Reiki for Beginners

Unlocking the Secrets of Reiki: A Step-by-Step Guide to Reiki Healing for Beginners to Achieve Physical and Spiritual Wellness

Caroline Kirkman

Table of Contents

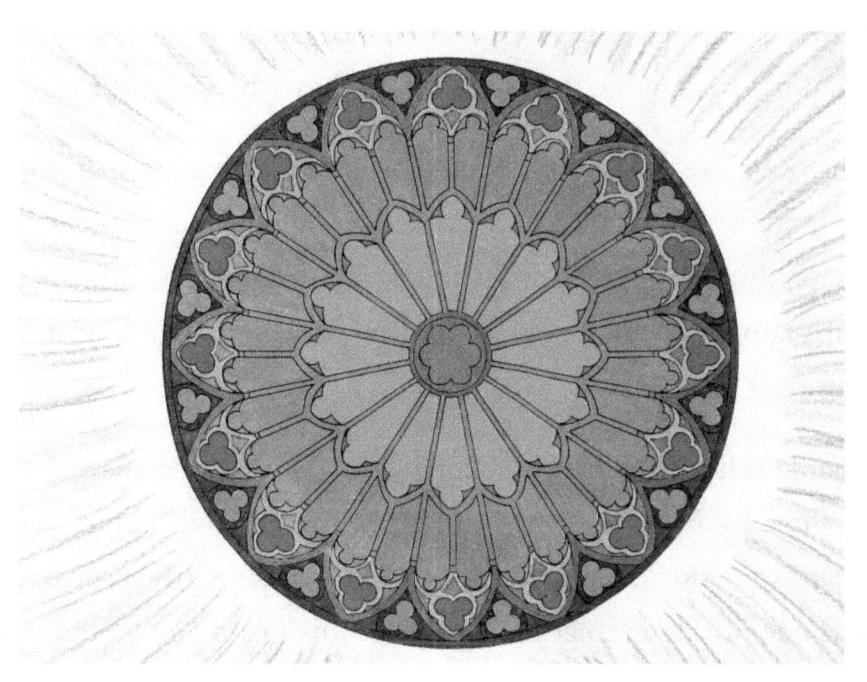

Introduction

Healing!

The word sums up the desires of many people in the world right now. Most people who want healing from something they are dealing with internally. However, the real question is, how can they get a long-term effect? It drives us to seek sustainable solutions, and at the top of the list, we have the answer: Reiki.

The Reiki story is unique. It speaks of a Japanese healing technique that aids in stress reduction and relaxation. It's generally administered by the laying of hands on the aching body part, supported by the concept of an unseen energy that flows within us.

People believe that if our life force is low, we become susceptible to illnesses or stress. When it is high, we can live a happy and healthy life. Reiki has helped many individuals with self-healing, but one of the fascinating aspects of this technique is that you can utilize it for distant healing. The practice entails sending energy across time and space to heal someone.

There is also a relationship between Reiki and chakras. Chakras are based on the concept of Yogi philosophy. They are like vortexes that aid the radiation of energy that corresponds with the physical body. Despite the presence of several chakras, the focus is always on the seven main ones as they emit light energy.

The purpose of Reiki is to heal and protect a person's body by striking a balance between their physical, mental, social, and emotional states. However, if a chakra is damaged or blocked, it will be unable to channel the energy in the right way. So, when they are balanced, they aid the successful transmission of the Reiki technique.

Nevertheless, this book isn't focused on chakras. Despite the connection between the two amazing methods, we will concentrate on Reiki and how you can use it to attain a good spiritual and physical well-being. For a more detailed insight into the relationship between the said techniques, you can get my book called *Chakras for Beginners, Healing Yourself With Chakras and Meditation. A Complete Guide to Third Eye and Chakra Healing for Starters With Practical Exercises to Balance Your Chakras.*

We are going to take on a journey towards healing profoundly and effectively. We will make several stops that will make up the entirety of the ideas from sections on how you can learn the practice of Reiki to the kind of ailments you may cure with this treatment. What you have in your hands is a complete Reiki guide that has been carefully put together to help you attain healing and more.

Are you ready to embark on this journey now? We will start with building a solid foundation on this topic with a detailed chapter on the Reiki story.

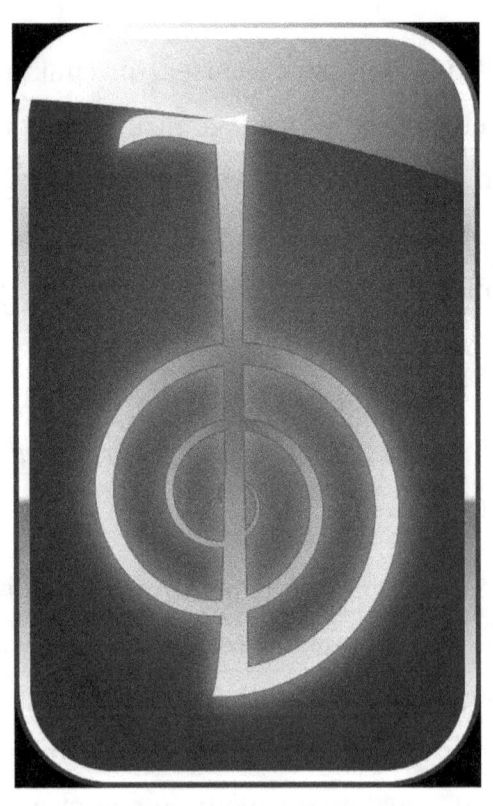

Chapter One: The Reiki Story

The first stop is a foundational one that entails complete details about the concept of Reiki. This chapter will provide insight into how the technique emerged, as well as the peculiarities of the process.

We'll cover a bit of the history of Reiki so that you can understand it better.

When you hear the word Reiki, you are listening to a combination of two Japanese words "Rei" and "Ki." Rei means a higher intelligence, God's wisdom, or higher power, while Ki refers to a spiritually guided life or non-physical energy that animates all living things.

The Reiki method of healing was established on the understanding of the body's energy system with a keen focus to restore balance. It was often used in self-care and offered in private practice and hospitals as a source of support therapy. It could be seen as a source of supportive therapy.

The form of Reiki practiced today has been in existence for over a hundred years. It began with Dr. Maiko Usui, the creator of the technique.

In modern usage of Reiki, you will discover a blend of medicine and psychology as these were the interests that drove Dr. Usui to seek ways to heal himself and others by the laying of hands. He wanted this practice to be accessible to everyone who needed healing.

So, how did Reiki become a global phenomenon from being a discovery that's made by one man?

After Dr. Usui's death, another doctor he had trained, Dr. Hayashi, took over in Tokyo and developed Reiki further by including the hand positions that could cover the body thoroughly. Dr. Hayashi also trained other Reiki maestros.

One of the Reiki masters, Mrs. Hawayo Takata, is a Japenese-American who got credited for bringing Reiki to the United States. Reiki saved Mrs. Takata from needing surgery. She enjoyed the process, found it helpful and relaxing, and gained more knowledge before bringing it to the states. Just like Dr. Hiyashi, Mrs. Takata also made some positive changes to the Reiki system. Before passing away, she trained 22 Reiki masters (International Association of Reiki Professionals, 2019).

The people who practice Reiki today use the methods that were developed by Dr. Usui. These practitioners can do that to heal themselves while enhancing their well-being. The modern Reiki masters can provide energy to other people through a gentle, light pressure using the Reiki hand position.

Since its inception, Reiki has been known to assist people who are dealing with diseases, pain, illnesses, and so on. You will learn more about the specific problems Reiki can solve in the fourth chapter.

Reiki is a non-physical healing energy that is guided by a higher intelligence or spiritually guided life force. Reiki is used to aid the body's natural healing abilities, reduce stress, and promote relaxation. This technique uses a hands-on approach as a way to transmit the unforeseen energy that flows from the practitioner to the patient.

Reiki is an intelligent energy that targets the area where healing is needed and restores harmony. Reiki practitioners assure that the treatment is bound to bring the required results as long as they follow the guides. They simply need to transmit life force into a recipient's body while focusing on key areas.

Today, many people have a backlog of physical issues they suppress. The reason is that they only concentrate on the surface of the problem, which is only a minute aspect of it. So, there are numerous ideas that become implemented to suppress the issue, which rises again occasionally because it hasn't been dealt with entirely.

With Reiki, the approach is different in a positive way. You get an opportunity to heal the source of the problem, not the symptoms. When you show up for a session, you should be ecstatic because you will get rid of your ailment once and for all.

If a person seeks out Reiki for a back issue, for example, the focus will not be on giving them relief but healing the source of the pain, thus removing the causes and effects of the problem entirely. Of course, the symptoms may not disappear immediately; however, with consistent Reiki sessions, healing will take place as time will prove to work on this.

Modern Reiki is gaining popularity just as the list of Reiki masters increases every day. People only become interested in becoming a master at something when they know it works for sure and that it will enable them to help others.

Reiki is also used in cancer clinics, spas, wellness centers, and hospitals. Some of them have a Reiki program in addition to other healing practices. Others stick with Reiki only because they are already convinced that it will yield the desired results.

Most professionals like to describe Reiki as a holistic healing system because it relates to the whole being and cuts across the physical, emotional, mental, and spiritual aspects of an individual. The body isn't viewed as a separate piece with different functions when doing Reiki. Instead, it is seen as a web of energy where everything works in agreement to provide balance for each part.

To attain good health, every aspect of the body has to be in tandem, and this is what Reiki tries to ensure. You need the continuous flow of life force to be healthy. Once there is an imbalance with this flow, you will start to experience negative emotions and health complications.

The masters of Reiki firmly believe that the universal energy is responsible for the bodily processes. This is the reason why every session will be about keeping that balance intact. Through the hands of the practitioner, the universal energy flows into the body of the receiver, which will aid in the healing procedure.

Reiki therapists often find clarity with their purpose in life because they notice that attending therapy consistently can boost their mindfulness through meditation, use of sacred symbols, precepts, and mantras that the practitioners can navigate through while performing hands-on healing.

Another fascinating thing about Reiki is that it doesn't cause any damage to the body. There is a lot of apprehension within individuals when they are offered a healing process that doesn't entail the use of drugs, surgery, or any other medical enabler. Their fears are real because no one wants to get hurt while trying to get healed, right? Well, if you are afraid of this practice, you should know that Reiki doesn't harm anyone who tries it.

Some Reiki masters say that they do not consider themselves as healers because they believe that the body is its own healer and that what they do is transmit the universal energy while the body does the rest of the work. Furthermore, they believe that the process of giving Reiki to someone else gives them more life energy. So, it is merely a case of giving extra power to do more and reawaken the positive vibes that make a person feel great about themselves again and enable healing.

We are swarmed by activities in the modern world; hence, we run around empty with just enough energy to go through what we can take for a day. This means that there is no more gas left for maintenance or more profound healing. When you offer your body universal energy, though, it uses this source for bodily repair.

If you are discovering Reiki now through this book, one thing you should know for sure is the fact that there are no limits to the possibilities it offers. If you look back at the brief history that we have just talked about, you will agree that the different changes and improvements made by each of the earliest Reiki masters indicate that the techniques and skills will always develop through time.

Reiki's energy comes from an infinite source. Even if the methods see innovation in the future, we will still be dealing with the same kind of energy that was used in the past. When a person meditates on Reiki's energy even when passing the treatment to others, they are aware of the positive essence that's embedded in the universal energy.

The latter goes beyond the state of consciousness and introduces the feeling of happiness, peace, and joy. These feelings are not just a figment of the imagination but a palpable experience that will help you achieve healing. People who have stayed true to the Reiki experience agree that as they get better, the practice not only helps them deal with their illnesses but also other issues.

In addition to healing from diseases, you will observe more positive traits with your personality when you start learning Reiki. However, in the beginning, you must identify your unhealthy features and become willing to let them go. After all, Reiki respects free will. When you accept the practice in your life, you must also surrender to its spiritual path, allow the process to heal you entirely, and develop the qualities that are healthy for you.

As your quality of life improve, you will notice that the more Reiki sessions you attend, the more deeply connected you become with your personality, emotions, and personal beliefs. All of them can contribute to your emotional well-being.

The first thing that you probably did after reading the title was to skimp through the Table of Contents because you wanted to find out what was in store for you in the actual chapters. Despite that, it is a good thing that you have taken a step towards learning by reading the actual content.

You may have read a sentence representing a chapter in the table, but here you are, reading more than three pages for that one sentence. Why? The reason is that the essence of greatness isn't defined by the introductory points. This idea is true for Reiki at least.

When you go to your first Reiki session, you may be looking forward to do some hands-on healing because that is what you have seen other masters do. However, you will also discover that there is so much to unearth about the process. You may even decide to go for a session because of physical or emotional pain that you have been dealing with silently and get healed from it.

So, I am not saying that Reiki is focused on one thing at a time, which makes it quite fascinating. Patience, non-competitiveness, self-love, and love for others are some of the positive, healthy traits you will start to develop after attending more profound sessions. If you have struggled with accepting others for who they are, you can also be sure that Reiki will help you move to a place of acceptance while gaining the power to forgive quickly.

Now, we will deliberate more on the benefits of Reiki in two other chapters, so we don't have to express such interests in detail here. With the use of Reiki comes the access to the energy flow it represents.

Have you ever gotten a library card before? If you had a library card, then you would know that it gives you access to all the books in the library. Still, it doesn't mean that you will read the entire collection of books that it houses.

Well, the same idea applies to Reiki. Through the first sessions you engage in, you will gain access to the universal energy. Will you get to channel the most effective qualities of Reiki, though? No. You have access to the energy just as you have done with your library card, so you need to utilize this privilege and build on the power that you have received by going for more sessions.

Like the situation with the library card, you may not be able to read all the books in there, but you can go through a large pile as long as you keep on going to the library and using the card. You will experience a higher level of peace, joy, and love during each session, which further opens you up to get healed through Reiki.

Regardless of what is written or said about Reiki, it is better to be experienced than heard. Like Mrs. Takata said, "I can't tell you, but I can show you."

Going forward from this chapter, you will only encounter practical ideas that will provide insight into the Reiki experience. The next section will give you details on how you can learn the practice, so enjoy reading!

Chapter Two: How to Learn Reiki

Welcome to the first chapter of the practical aspect of our journey. Now that you know the theoretical points of the subject matter, we will take you through a series of steps that you can utilize to learn how to practice Reiki.

As it was clearly stated in the previous chapter, there are higher levels of universal energy. We may not be able to take on all of them because it requires a lot of training, but what you will receive here is a solid foundation and a good start for your Reiki practice.

The system that you will be exposed to is the same one used by Dr. Mikao Usui. Through this system, you will experience amazing improvements in your personal, emotional, and spiritual well-being. You can also observe changes in the lives of the people you share this process with. Hence, it is a great way to introduce Reiki into your relationships.

The variants of Reiki have been used worldwide by holy men, healers, and Rishis. They used to believe that everything in the world was made up of vibrational energy. The system also works because it improves the energetic make-up of the body, which makes it possible for the root causes of the problem to be handled.

When you heal with Reiki, three things can happen to you:

1. Your body's energetic blueprints are improved.

2. Your body adopts the new state causing much healing.

3. You can tap into the universal energy flow.

The first step that you can take towards the mastery of Reiki is your choice to focus on the entirety of your system while inviting the grace to heal, clear all the mental barriers in your head, and believe in the efficacy of the steps that will be shared below.

Please remember that this is a practical chapter. You must read everything carefully because you can use them to apply Reiki healing into your life.

Steps for Learning Reiki

Step 1: Connect With the Universal Energy

Universal energy is the building block for reality, and it is everywhere. It explains the discovery made by scientists that the universal energy field genuinely exists all around us. Reiki healers tap into this energy pool and then channel it to provide life-changing benefits for us and their patients.

For you to tap into the universal energy, your consciousness needs to increase to a higher level where you can tune yourself into the realities that exist beyond the physical world — a realm of emotions, love, thoughts, and heightened spirituality.

Some people are always skeptical of this first step because they erroneously believe that they don't have the "gift" to form this secure connection with the energy source. Well, those Reiki masters who have access to the highest forms dedicated their lives to studying and practicing. If you have the diligence and determination to settle with each step and practice for a long time, you will surely have a success story to tell. But first, you must handle this initial stage before perfecting the others.

Step #1 entails that you must make a connection with the universal energy, which has a consciousness. To begin this process, you must clear your mind and ask for permission to be used as a healing channel first.

Speak the Reiki invocation out loud or think about it. The words have to be in line with your beliefs. You can say simple words, such as "I ask the power and wisdom of universal energy to allow me to become a channel for infinite love and healing..."

The invocation above is just an example. You can create yours, but the point is that you need to ask the universal energy for its help so that it can channel its gift to you. By acknowledging that you need assistance, you will be giving up any claim you may have had in the past to the power of your own.

Next, you need to visualize the energy entering your palms. Visualization is so powerful because it allows you to connect with the energy (you will observe as we make progress that visualization cuts across almost all the steps). There are numerous visualization processes that will help you connect with universal Energy, but you can utilize the one that's known as INFINITE LIGHT:

- Close your eyes and breathe in.

- Exhale and visualize the beams of white energy all around you.

- Feel the energy from its infinite field.

- Inhale and when you exhale this time focus on your palms while using your will to call on the light around you.

- Visualize the light entering your body and flowing into your palms.

- Feel your palms as they radiate energy.

The most critical part of this step isn't getting every aspect of it right but feeling the energy, and this is what a lot of people haven't got right. By practicing the concept of universal energy visualization, you will be able to feel and sense it all around you.

When you visualize the connection taking place, you will be focused on your will that makes the link happen and then your thoughts, willpower and everything else that comes in contact with this energy flow will cause the Reiki reality to take shape.

You have a grasp on how to get in touch with universal energy. The next step will teach you how to detect negative energy present in your body.

Step 2: Perform an Aura Scan

An aura is a form of universal energy that surrounds objects and living things, but you may be surprised to know that your body does not give off an aura because it is an overlay on it. To put it simply, you are not giving off an aura, but your aura is giving off you.

So, your aura puts off and absorbs information. It is a part of your energy system that can transmit and receive signals. Auras have different properties that cut across, sizes, patterns, textures, shapes, and colors.

All of your memories, emotions, thoughts, and experiences exist in your aura, and this plays a crucial role in affecting your health. Your body is a physical representation of your aura, and your physical health is also dependent on the health of your aura.

To explain the connection between your aura and your health, you've got to think back to when you harbored specific negative thoughts in your mind and how it affected you. In such moments, it starts to show up in your aura as a dark muddy clot, which then takes the shape of a physical symptom.

Whatever you feel is a manifestation of your aura. If you feel pain, are depressed, or have problems with your relationship, then it is safe to say they manifest from your aura. This feeling helps you realize what needs to be done to bring it back to a beneficial state enough to result in healing for the symptoms.

This second step requires you to be able to tell the areas of your aura that has problems and how you can sense the circumstances that led to the aura being the exact way it is now.

However, scanning your aura can be a worthless pursuit if you don't understand the life force optimization system, which is required to serve as a map for healing using high sensory perception and feelings with the hands.

When you become conscious of your aura, it will directly lead you to the next step of the process through which you can learn Reiki, and that step entails setting your healing intentions.

Step 3: Realize Your Healing Intention

This step and the previous ones will show you how to heal the underlying energetic problems that are responsible for the physical symptoms you experience.

Your healing intention is the result you would like to experience from the healing sessions. Do you remember going to the gym at any time, for instance? What were your expectations? Did you want better abs? A right waistline or a flat stomach?

The expectations you had when you registered for the gym helped to keep you accountable. This is the same with this third step. Regardless of what you want healing for, maybe an injury, a more positive emotional state or to find balance in your life, you must have healing expectations.

Your intention is your message!

When you send a message to your friend, you are communicating something to the person. However, with Reiki, the message is not received by the person who is going to be healed but by their aura.

If the message is clear and precise, the aura will accept it and transform it to match the positive message you are sending them. The aura then projects the new and improved state to the body.

You cannot have a Reiki session without an intention. Your healing plan tells the aura the form it should take. This means that before your session, you must spend time alone to discover what you seek healing from. Say, do you want to get over a trauma, improve your sleep, or overcome addiction?

The aura will only accept a dominant healing intention as this kind of intention can lead to a life-changing healing process that blossoms into reality, thus relieving you of the issues.

Again, with this step, you will have to rely on a Reiki process we introduced with the first step: visualization! With visualization, you can manifest your desires. Just imagine what your life would be like if you didn't have the challenge you are dealing with.

You should ask yourself what your life will be like without the pain and then try to visualize the answer. Imagine yourself healed and create vivid images in the mind of your healing intention coming to fruition.

If you want to use Reiki for back pain that has deprived you of dancing, for instance, don't go for the healing session focusing on the back pain. Instead, think about the kind of music you want to dance to once you are healed, visualize it, and take advantage of the positivity it brings.

Visualize the tissues in your back getting healed and the pain going away. This is how you set your healing intentions and work on rebuilding yourself to attain the healing you desire. Have you heard about Reiki symbols? Well, it is about time you discovered what they are and what you can do with them.

Step 4: Activate Reiki Symbols

Reiki symbols help you tune yourself to a particular level of frequencies that give you access to advanced abilities. The symbols have been used for generations, and they are fully imbibed with energy from great healers over the years.

In learning how to practice Reiki, you must choose the symbols you wish to utilize, and your decision is based on the abilities you desire to use. For example, you can use the mental and emotional symbol for issues relating to relationship challenges or an addiction.

So, what are the Reiki symbols?

The Power Symbol

This symbol can magnify healing energy and provide spiritual protection while empowering other symbols. The power symbol is known as *Cho Ku Rei.*

The Master Symbol

The Master symbol is the most potent symbol in Reiki that is used by the masters to heal a soul or treat illness and diseases in the body, thus creating a fantastic life change for the individual. The Master symbol is referred to as *Di KoMyo.*

The Distance Symbol

The Distance symbol is a unifying one that represents enlightenment and peace. The symbol is also used to send healing energy over distance and time to anyone who is in the past, present, or future. The Distance symbol is also known as *Hon Sha ZeShoNen.*

The Mental and Emotional Symbol

This symbol is tuned to the energies of love and well-being while being used for restoring calm to a person's mental and emotional states. The mental and emotional symbols can also be useful in removing addictions and releasing negative energies from a person. The Mental and Emotional symbol is also known as *Sei He Ki.*

Everything in the system and the steps you are following work harmoniously to transform your life through the universal energy. Regardless of where you are now or what your issues may be, you are dealing with the Reiki symbols that can be used to manifest the changes you seek.

What are you struggling with? Drugs, alcohol, emotional pain? All of these can change when you start allowing the universal energy into your life. Express gratitude while on this path, especially after activating the symbols mentioned above.

With these symbols, you can transmit healing energy into the areas of your body in need of a cure. Discover how to do this in the next step.

Step 5: Guide Healing Energy

Now, this fifth step is a culmination of all the other steps you read through up till this point. You may know that, as a healer, your hands can be positioned correctly to guide energy into the aura and chakras that need healing.

Despite that, the hand positions will not work by themselves. You need to manifest the healing by creating a secure connection with steps 1 to 4.

These steps, when used together, lay the foundation for your healing session and enable you to channel energy and use it for the right purpose. With the hand positions alone and a weak energy connection, you may be able to get a small amount of healing, but you can get so much more combining all the steps. You can harness the potential that lies within Reiki and allow it to manifest the changes you desire in your well-being.

So, this is how you can become better with Reiki: by using the system created by these steps to aid the realization of your healing intention. After laying the right foundation, you can then go further with aura cleansing, reiki breath, chakra balancing, etc.

With step 3, you set your healing intentions and formal message that is sent to your aura. This message details the kind of positive changes you want to see, and you transmit it by guiding the universal energy to your will.

While on the process, if you discover other issues while going about your aura scan, repeat steps 3 to 6 until the issues are taken off.

Now, you are going to learn how to close your Reiki connection safely with the next step.

Step 6: Close Your Connection

Reiki sessions shouldn't end without you taking this step. Reiki masters say that while they work with patients, they absorb the negative emotions of the patient and feel it lodged in their system.

You should ensure that the emotions are released from your body so that you can continue to enjoy a heightened state of energy. Again, you will have to rely on visualization to get this done by visualizing the energies being pulled out of your body through your palms and freeing your system.

Wash your hands afterwards in cold water, so they are purified and ensure that all residual energies are out entirely. Also, ensure that you are not in any way attached to the healing session emotionally. Believe that the energy is gone and take the last step below.

Step 7: Expand Your Energy Channels

Now, you have to consistently increase the channeling of your energy in between sessions so that your healing ability can be better in terms of effectiveness. This way, you will also be able to perform advanced techniques and progress to higher Reiki levels.

So, how can you expand your energy channels?

Firstly, you can utilize Ki exercises, which are meditations that you can practice by cycling energy through your system. These exercises open your chakras to allow more universal energy to get into your body and channeled towards healing.

Secondly, you can use attunements, which help you become harmonious with something. It is the primary way of advancing from the level of Reiki you are already in to another one. Attunement is like a radio dial; you only get a station when you turn into its frequency.

Most people can practice the primary forms of Reiki, so you need these exercises to be able to go over and beyond the fundamental level.

There will never be a better time to discover true happiness that happens as a result of the alignment you attain with your higher self. You know yourself best, you know the challenges you encounter daily, so if you want to experience some peace,now is the time to get on with Reiki healing.

You can use the ideas proffered in this chapter to embark on the most profound healing experience that will enable you to define your existence and live to your most accurate potentials.

Still, how does a Reiki session work? Do you know all about the positions of the hand and how distant Reiki treatment is done? To get answers to these questions and more, please flip over to the next chapter.

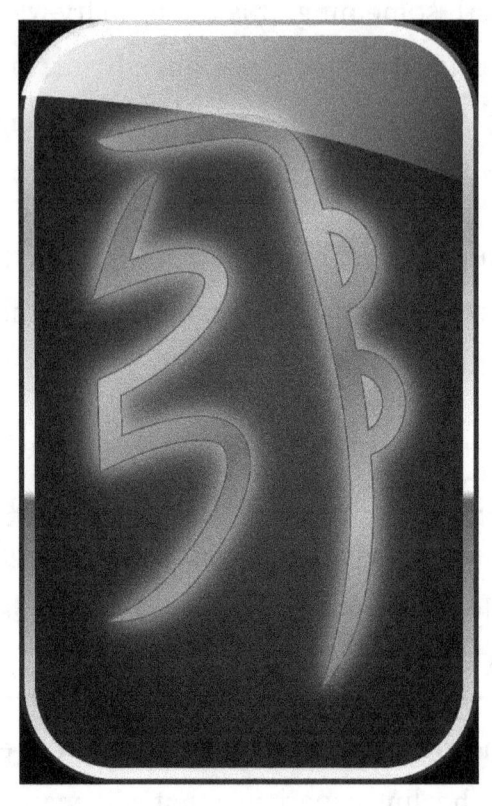

Chapter Three: How a Reiki Session Works

A Reiki session is quite an exciting experience because there are no typical sessions, set protocols, or length of time for all of them. Reiki healing can also be administered by anyone who has gone through training.

Healthcare providers, family members, or even you, after getting training, can use it to help someone else. There are also no typical settings for a Reiki session, although a quiet place is preferable.

Some people feel anxious about their Reiki session beforehand because, regardless of what they have read online or in books, they believe that nothing will ever prepare them for it than the experience itself. So, the objective of this chapter is to provide insight into how a Reiki session works so that you get an idea of the entire proceedings, know what to expect, and look forward to it with positive optimism.

You will also learn more about the traditional positions of hands, as well as the concept of self and distant Reiki healing.

For you to have a great experience, it is advised to choose a Reiki practitioner or friend who is well-trained at it and somehow you are comfortable with. It is crucial to feel good vibes with this person because, as you know, the universal energy cannot be forced.

The person you settle for should first describe the process and how he or she will structure the session to give you an idea of what to expect. Knowing what the individual will do next will be instrumental in keeping you relaxed and helping you build trust.

A Reiki session should take place in a quiet place where you wouldn't be disturbed or distracted. The professional Reiki practitioners have a dedicated space they use, and some may want to play instrumental music to mask out any noisy interference, but you can speak up if you prefer a silent room.

If you are going to receive Reiki in a hospital or nursing home, then it is possible that your session will be a shorter one (between 15 to 20 minutes). If you are taking the meeting in private, you can get up to 90 minutes per session (the time varies at the discretion of the practitioner's choice).

Now, what about the actual process? For some practitioners, an intake form is a part of their session as they use it to carry out a health interview, especially if the practitioner has some background training in health care or other forms of therapy. Meanwhile, others believe that Reiki is a form of folk practice instead of a healthcare solution; hence, they avoid using an intake form. For both types of practitioners, though, you may be required to sign a consent form, which is part of the standard practice.

After signing the consent or intake form, the professional will ask you some questions that give him or her insight into your specific needs while explaining the process. At this stage, being honest about how you feel is the surest way of getting the best out of the remaining part of the session.

So, try not to skip anything and be as transparent as you can by letting the professional know your needs, health conditions that you have been dealing with, and every other information that will give the practitioner more clarity regarding your case.

If you are taking the Reiki session in the hospital, the therapist may ask your permission to touch the painful areas as you explain. After this step, they will signal you to get ready for the session itself.

You will be required to lay on a table, fully clothed, or sit in a chair. Reiki will be offered through light touch that is non-invasive, with the practitioner's hand placed on the painful part of your body, as well as several other locations like your back, torso, head, etc. The placement of the practitioner's hand shouldn't be inappropriate or have too much pressure.

Moreover, there can be additional placements on your limbs if you have an old injury that still hurts. The practitioner can also hold their hands over an open wound or a burn as it is a way of offering Reiki to that injury. While all of this is going on, you may be wondering how you will be feeling or what you will experience during the sessions.

Some patients said that they felt refreshed or that they could think clearer in those moments. Others mentioned feeling like they were in a spa. Instead of a spa for the physical body, though, they were in a resort for the mind. At some point, you may feel like you are falling asleep or experience the same relaxed sensation that you get after a rewarding activity. These are some of the feelings people express during a Reiki session. Remember, it varies from one person to another.

Reiki experience is entirely subjective and often changeable. While it may be subtle for one person, it may be a fascinating experience for another person. Some people say they experience heat from the palms of the practitioner, which signals the flow of energy. For others, the practitioner's palms are relaxed. Another simplified Reiki session experience is that the patient feels subtle energy pulses as the practitioner's hands move over certain areas.

However, there is one feeling that cuts across most Reiki patients, and it is the feeling of comfort as recipients testify that they often feel like they are between the thresholds of consciousness (still being aware of their surroundings) and a sleep-like state that makes them as if they are meditating, even though they are not.

I know you probably think that there truly is a myriad of emotional experiences, and it all makes Reiki exciting and dramatic at the same time. With your first session, you may not get all of these feelings at once, but you will surely feel some release of stress and a sense of relaxation that makes you feel like you should come for another session.

Still, what's most interesting is the fact that, even after the session, you are bound to feel great afterwards. If you take on another meeting, your body gets used to it, and you can improve your aura while getting healed from the issues you have had.

The truth about Reiki is that it is mostly cumulative. Even if you don't feel anything at the beginning or with your first session, it doesn't dispute the fact that something has taken place within your body. It has been proven that people who do not get a mix of all of these experiences at first tend to have more profound experience later if they continue with the sessions.

Other notable changes that may consistently take place includes a sense of being poised, high reactivity, and better connection with the universe.

So, what should you do during the session?

After finding a great practitioner whom you are comfortable with, during the sessions, you can do a series of things, such as coming with the music you enjoy so that you can relax with familiar music while the expert does his or her work.

You can also use the restroom before the session so that you can lay comfortably without interruptions. If you are shy about being touched, ask the practitioner to show you the areas that he or she will reach during the meeting so that you can be mentally prepared and feel comfortable before it happens.

If you have trouble breathing while lying down, let the practitioner know before the session starts. If you had surgery, inform them about it as well so that they can float their hands over it or touch it tenderly. Pregnant women should also mention their condition before the session commences. For people who have digestive complaints, they may also have difficulty lying on their stomach, so the practitioner should be aware of it.

You will feel more relaxed during the session when the Reiki professional knows everything that they should know about you. You can ask for anything that will make you feel even more comfortable, such as a blanket or support under your knees. The practitioner will be there for you to make the process seamless and enjoyable for you.

When you start the session, don't just try to relax. Instead, do it for real.

Reiki is mostly a passive experience when the session starts as most of the work is done by the practitioner. At this point, you only need to enjoy the process and do nothing else.

Diagnosis is not a part of Reiki sessions when you are done with the practitioner. Nevertheless, some practitioners may have suggestions for you on following your body's needs, drinking more water, etc. Some people say that they leave a Reiki session feeling refreshed and then very tired afterward, and this is just the body's reaction to the natural healing process. On the evening of your first session, you will feel a sense of calm, have a good night sleep, and operate with mental clarity.

The number of sessions you are meant to have subsequently is determined by the practitioner, who may suggest a series of sessions afterward. The traditional recommendation is four sessions as it gives you ample opportunity to evaluate your benefits. You can discuss with the practitioner the ways through which you can spread the session to suit your needs or peculiar schedule.

If you have a very serious health condition, for instance, the practitioner may recommend that you take on four sessions in four consecutive days. However, you can choose to take it all as an advice and do what's best for you.

The Traditional Positions of the Hands

There cannot be a complete discourse on the impact and practice of Reiki without talking about the conventional positions of the hands. The hands are the medium through which energy flows. For any Reiki session to become successful, the practitioner must apply the right-hand usage for the right situation. There are several traditional hand positions, and we will take the time to present most of them later so that you can get acquainted with the motions that aid with Reiki success.

Below, you will gain access to 12 hand positions.

First Position: The Face

With this position, the hands are placed over the recipient's face, with the palms gently positioned on the forehead and fingers cupped tenderly over the eyes.

The position also allows the recipient to keep on breathing freely because the airways will be open as the practitioner ensures that there are no constrictions with the nose during the session.

Second Position: The Crown and Top of the Head

The wrist plays a pivotal role in this hand position as the practitioner uses the inner wrist to wrap his or her hands around the recipient's head. The fingertips will touch the ears for a more extensive feel.

Third Position: The Back of the Head

Here, the practitioner's hands will be gently tucked under the recipient's head while forming a cradle for the head. The back of the practitioner's hand will relax and rest on the table.

Fourth Position: Chin and Jawline

With this position, you get to surround the recipient's jawline with your hands while allowing your fingertips to touch underneath the chin and the heels of your hand near the recipient's ears.

Fifth Position: Neck, Collarbone, and Heart

While the patient is lying down, you will wrap your right hand lightly under his or her neck. If the recipient is uncomfortable with it, allow your hand to hover above the neck only. Then, stretch your left arm downwards and place your hand at the center of the heart.

Sixth Position: Ribs and Rib Cage

This hand position requires you to place your hand on the upper rib cage. Ensure that it is below the breast, though, because you are not supposed to touch private areas when treating someone, even if it's accidental.

Seventh Position: Abdomen

The practitioner's hand should be placed on the stomach, above the recipient's navel, close to the solar plexus area.

Eighth Position: Pelvic Bones

You need to place both palms over each pelvic bone.

Ninth Position: Shoulder Blades

Here, you will have to help the recipient change position from being on his or her back to lying on the stomach. Then, place your hands on the shoulder blades because it is a region that has a lot of emotional burdens. You have to keep your palms on the position longer so that you can dislodge the stuck energies.

Tenth Position: Mid-Back

The practitioner should place his or her hands on the middle area of the recipient's back.

Eleventh Position: Lower Back

Still on the back, you will use the hand position to get to the recipient's lower back region.

Twelfth Position: Sacrum

When the session is complete, the practitioner combs the recipient's aura with his or her hands to ensure that all energetic debris is cleared out. This debris may have come from the physical body during the session.

Also, you can make a silent request to the universe, saying that all negative energies should be transformed into positive ones!

We are still discovering more about how Reiki works, and we will be taking it a step further by learning how you can use Reiki as a self-treatment. It promises to be a fascinating sub-section, so keep on reading.

How Reiki Self-Treatment Works

Using self-treatment is an essential aspect of the Reiki healing program. If you can set aside 15 to 30 minutes daily to administer Reiki to yourself, you will be able to achieve a whole lot with your physical, emotional, and mental well-being.

Reiki self-treatment isn't different from the one done between a practitioner and a recipient as you will be utilizing your hand positions as well. When giving yourself Reiki, your vibration will go up, making it the perfect time for you to achieve all you set out to do in your life. You will also discover new habits, attitudes, creative ideas, and solutions on how you can handle life's pressing issues.

There are numerous ways to practice Reiki, but all of these, regardless of the variants, must be done practically. After all, Reiki is never done in the abstract. If you settle for a system that works for yourself, it will become easier for you to practice daily, get better at it, and make it a part of your life.

Before you decide on doing Reiki self-treatment, you must seek out the challenges you are having and have an honest discussion with yourself about them, just like you would do with a practitioner. Armed with information on what you need help with, you can take on the path towards self-treatment and get a cure.

You can start with self-practice by concentrating on these critical areas: throat, lower rib, navel, back of the head, the crown of the head, face, throat, and lower abdomen. You can lay on your side with a pillow, doubled over, and then stay on your back to get it done.

Your practice time should be synchronized with your schedule. Don't just stick to anyone's schedule that you have seen online; seek out what works for you instead and use it. If it is in the morning, then you should do it as soon as you wake up before opening your eyes.

Let your hands spread to the parts of your body that you want to work with. As you savor the energy, allow yourself to be drawn into the experience. At the end of your sessions, linger a bit in bed to complete it, then wash your hands and drink lots of water before embarking on your day.

Organize Your Practice

If you like to have intervals in between, that's your choice as well. You can use a timer to signal the breaks you will take or download Reiki timer apps on your mobile device. Also, introduce a protocol to your self-treatment as it helps your hand to create a habit of doing so without thinking. The more you practice, the more natural it becomes for your hand positions.

Remember to prop yourself up in a very comfortable position as well so that you are not focused on your body but your experience. Don't rely on random times during the day to practice or when the chosen time comes to use your hand positions to administer healing.

Now, there will be days when it feels like you cannot be

consistent. Don't beat yourself up about it and ensure that you are not putting too much pressure on yourself. Instead of rushing for 30 to 40 minutes to practice the routine, you can start with 10 minutes and gradually build it up. After all, a little practice is better than none at all.

Use the pattern: Practice-observe-contemplate-repeat!

How Distant Reiki Treatment Works

A lot of people are unsure about the concept of remote Reiki sessions, and it is easy to understand their skepticism because one can only marvel at the possibility of being able to transfer healing to someone else in another place through this process. How can someone else in another room, city, or country experience heal from a Reiki practitioner, right?

Well, we have already established the fact that Reiki uses healing energy, and it cannot be contained or confined to a room. Within our material world, we must do everything in person, e.g., go shopping, walk the dog, etc. However, these are physical activities that are made through the body, and they do not make use of Reiki.

Reiki can be holistically used to restore the balance to a person's body, mind, and spirit. It can also promote the regenerative abilities of the universal energy because it goes beyond the physical. We have the power inside our body, and this energy has its vibrations, which creates a field around us, a.k.a. the energy field.

Four Fields of Energy

Energy fields can be felt through touch. This is the reason why Reiki is performed with the hands.

We have the emotional field, which is where we feel. It extends from 1 to 3 inches from the physical body.

There is the physical field, which is the first layer. It stays ¼ to 2 inches from the body.

We also have the mental field that is known for aiding our mental processes and thoughts. It can be sensed at 3 to 8 inches from the body.

The spiritual field consists of about four or more layers, helps us stay attuned to our spiritual reality, and extends by 6 to 20 inches beyond the body.

How to Do Distance Healing

You will use the energy fields to send healing to someone else in another place, and they will receive it. However, how can you do that?

First, you must ensure that your hands and chakras are empowered with the Power symbol. Then, you need to apply

Reiki to yourself for about 10 to 15 minutes. Next, you will need to invoke the distance healing symbols (remember what we discussed on symbols) and say the person's name three times.

While repeating their name, visualize the individual whom you want to send healing to and get ready to send the universal energy to each of their field levels.

If you want to send energy to a person's physical level, for instance, start by imagining it entering their chakra and then going inside their body and gently filling them up. As it happens, the organs in their bodies are also getting the vibration. Then, the energy starts to radiate. You see them glow with this energy and expand it as the different fields are full.

After sending healing to their physical field, you should also do the same to their emotional area next. You can do this by imagining them getting filled with so much joy, peace, satisfaction, and great well-being. Visualize the glow from their physical field getting into the emotional field.

Then, you can send universal energy to their mental field by intending for their thoughts to be very calm. They know what to do because their brain is working and the ideas are flowing smoothly. Now, imagine that they are getting solutions to their problems, believe that they are no longer worried, and Reiki is filling them up with high energy for their mental field.

Next, you will have to send energy to their spiritual field by visualizing it filling up their spirit and causing restoration. Visualize a renewal of their soul, mind, and essence as the flow of energy remains the direct link from where they are to heaven.

Your intention should be for them to be filled with spiritual energy beyond their being. As they feel everything, they should be able to embrace this new spiritual height that will transform their lives.

Now, before you do all of these, you must have a conversation with the individual who needs help. To be precise, ask them questions about each level and intentionally learn more about their challenges.

Don't ask vague questions; be direct by starting with each field. You can get to know how the patients are feeling emotionally if they are happy or sad to gain access to their emotional area. Then, try to find out if they have any pain in their bodies for the physical field.

Are they worried about something? Are they restless when sleeping? These are questions for the mental field. Ask them how their spirit feels and if they feel unsafe in the world as well for their spiritual field.

The fact that you know their issues doesn't mean that you get to perform Reiki immediately, though. Start by preparing them for it. Tell them to get ready for healing and that they should allow the universal energy to heal them. Then, you can do it for 10 to 20 minutes on each field level.

When the session is over, tell them to rest and visualize the Power symbol over them. Disconnect from their energy field by dry bathing, give yourself a few minutes of Reiki, and call them afterward to know how they are doing and what they have experienced. Always end all distant Reiki sessions with gratitude for the healing process.

Distant Reiki healing became very popular and essential when people realized that they didn't have to go through the stress of traveling from one country to another to get help. The time spent trying to book an appointment or meet a practitioner could be channeled into other productive things instead. More importantly, distant Reiki makes it possible for the recipient to be comfortable at home.

Some people may not feel free in an office or a Reiki space far from home. When they get the freedom to do it in their place, therefore, it adds a lot of value to the process for them. One-on-one sessions can also be much more expensive than distant healing.

So, getting Reiki from a distance is an excellent alternative to having a one-on-one session, which can be a source of inconvenience to a lot of people. Most individuals who have never practiced distant Reiki often end up preferring it after experiencing it for the first time because they get the same results as though they were in the same room with the practitioner.

Nonetheless, the only way to know if it works for you is to try it out yourself. Make sure it is scheduled for a time that you prefer and that you are in a quiet place, focused and ready to receive healing.

With distant Reiki, you don't have to work around someone else's schedule. You can also record the details of your healing while taking note of what works in which field, as well as what areas need more work.

Reiki sessions are the connecting dots between you and the healing you anticipate. As such, being prepared for it is essential. We have used this chapter to provide concise information that will prepare you for the Reiki sessions. While you may be looking forward to everything mentioned here in terms of the experience, you should know that no two sessions are the same.

Keep an open mind, enjoy the process, and love the experience it brings as this is the only way you can have a personalized Reiki experience! We are moving on to one of the most exciting parts of our journey as it deals with a question most people can't stop asking, "What ailment or disease can Reiki cure?"

Let's find out in the next section, shall we?

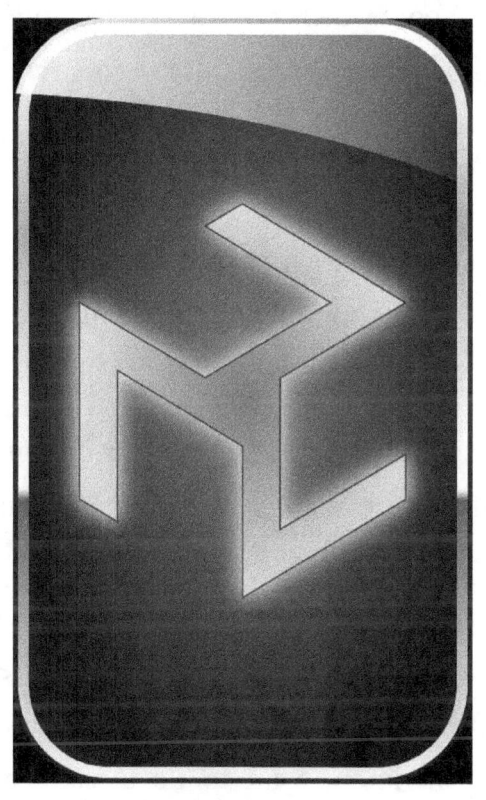

Chapter Four: Ailments Healed
With Reiki

One of the reasons why there is a lot of emphasis on Reiki treatment in the world today is that there are more success stories shared about their impact. Hence, many people are willing to not only give it a try but also become consistent with it.

Now, if you have never tried Reiki before, and this book is your first encounter with the subject matter, you would want to know the benefits you stand to gain by adopting this approach. After all, there are so many options available online, so one can only wonder what's so special about Reiki.

If you have practiced Reiki in the past or had prior knowledge about this healing process, then you must be curious to unearth the actual illnesses and diseases that Reiki can cure. This chapter will show you the types of conditions that can be treated with Reiki and explain how you can achieve the desired results with proper hand positions. We already covered the aspect of self-treatment, so you know what to do already if you want to administer it to yourself.

Not all Reiki sessions or treatment patterns are suitable for all diseases and illnesses. Before embarking on a treatment process, therefore, you will need to know the specific condition you are dealing with, as well as the kind of session and hand position to use. Let's discuss that briefly before getting right on to the types of illnesses that Reiki can cure.

There are specific positions of the entire body treatment with Reiki that is meant for specific symptoms. Such positions can be used for a longer time during the healing process. For such complaints, you only require quick yet consistent sessions. For example, chronic illnesses can be cured after four consecutive sessions. If there will be an extension, the seriousness of the disease will determine it.

Others may take a while before achieving immediate healing, primarily if we are talking about cancer in which weekly meetings may be required. The recipient will have to be patient and ensure that there is enough connection with all Reiki sessions for maximum effect.

For diseases that cause disfiguration of the body, the recipient will need to balance his or her second and fifth chakras. If they are dealing with life-threatening illnesses, they will have to focus on the fifth and sixth chakras.

If a person is dealing with paralysis or a form of impairment, then he or she should work on balancing the first, third, and fifth chakras. Reiki treatments are useful for illnesses that involve the nervous system and the mind.

Most importantly, you must know that Reiki treatment is not a substitute for consultation with a physician. It is not an alternative for psychotherapy or natural therapy sessions either.

If you find that you are increasingly worried about your state and you cannot stick to Reiki sessions, then you must consult a medical practitioner or visit a hospital.

Different Illnesses Reiki Treatment Can Cure

Please note that all solutions proffered below are also presented with the kind of hand positions that you can use to achieve the desired results. It isn't all about placing your hands on a person's body; you must transfer universal energy. If you are the recipient, the practitioner will do the same.

Now, the reason why most diseases are listed together in one section is that ailments and the Reiki treatment required have similar hand positions.

Headache and Backache

With headaches, one position doesn't apply for all at once, so you can try everything and stick to whichever is most effective.

First Position

The first step is to place your hand in a parallel position from the forehead to the region of the top teeth and then to the right and left of the nose.

Second Position

The practitioner's hands should cup the back of the recipient's head with his or her fingertips placed on the medulla oblongata. This is the soft spot along the midline of the head to the neck and halfway to where the hard bone ends and changes into a soft depression.

Third Position

The healer's hands should be placed between the shoulders and shoulder blades.

Fourth Position

The hands should remain on the shoulder blades at this point.

Fifth Position

The hands should then be on the soles of the feet. Specifically, the big toes have to be covered from the tips.

Backache

You can add local backache treatment to the hand Reiki positions below.

First Position

The practitioner should place his or her hands in a parallel position from the forehead to top teeth region and then to the right and left of the nose.

Second Position

The hands should now be on the shoulders and shoulder blades.

Third Position

Place the hands on the shoulder blades.

Fourth Position

The hands should cover the hollows of the knees.

Fifth Position

The hands should then be on the soles of the recipient's feet. Specifically, the big toes have to be covered from the tips.

Kidney and Liver Problems

First Position

The healer should place hands in a parallel position from the forehead to the region of the top teeth in an identical position to the right and left of the nose.

Second Position

The balls of the thumbs should be on the ridges of the pelvic bones. The tips of the hands should be close to each other at the pubic bone, forming a V.

Third Position

Place the hands on the lower ribs, right above the kidney.

Fourth Position

Place one hand on the sacral plate and the other one vertically below it with little pressure.

Fifth Position

Place the hands around the ankles.

Liver Complaints

First Position

One hand should be placed on the lowest ribs (right side) with another hand below it.

Second Position

Place one hand above the navel. Keep the other hand underneath it.

Third Position

Place the hands on the shoulder blades.

Arthritis, Pain, and Fractures

Arthritis

First Position

The hands of the healer should be on the lower ribs, above the kidney.

Second Position

The hands should then be on the soles of the feet. Specifically, the big toes have to be covered from the tips.

Pain

First Position

Place your hands between the shoulders and shoulder blades.

Second Position

The hands should now be placed on the shoulder blades. If the patient is complaining about bone pain, one hand should be put above and below the main cervical vertebra at the neck's nape.

If it is a pain in the hips and legs, the universal energy should be channeled to the entire back and outside the hips.

For arm pain, Reiki can be applied to the top of the shoulder with the positions below.

First Position

The hands should be placed between the shoulders and shoulder blades.

Second Position

The hands should stay on the shoulder blades.

Fractures

Reiki treatment needs to be performed regularly after the bones are set up with the hand positions below.

First Position

The practitioner should place one hand from the forehead to the region of the top teeth in a parallel position to the right and left of the nose.

Second Position

One hand should be placed gently on the lowest ribs and another one directly below it.

Third Position

With one hand on the sacral plate, the other hand should be placed vertically below with a little more pressure.

Fourth Position

The healer should place hands on the soles of the feet with the big toes covered from the tips.

Diabetes, Asthma, and Heart Attack

Diabetes

For Reiki treatment with diabetes, the elbows should receive a lot of concentration with the positions below.

First Position

The healer should place hands from the forehead to the region of the top teeth in a parallel position to the right and left sides of the nose.

Second Position

Hands should be placed on the left lower ribs and below it.

Third Position

The healer should place one hand across the thymus while the other hand is at a right angle below and between the breasts, forming a T.

Fourth Position

The hands are placed at the soles of the feet with the big toes covered from the tips.

Asthma

First Position

The healer's hands should cup the back of the recipient's head with fingertips place don the Medulla oblongata.

Second Position

The practitioner should place his or her hands in a parallel position to the right and the left of the nose. This should be done from the forehead to the region of the top teeth.

Third Position

With one hand placed across the thymus, the other hand should be at the right angle and between the breasts, forming a T.

Fourth Position

Place the balls of the thumb on the ridges of the pelvic bone with the tips of the hands close to each other at the pubic bone, forming a V.

Heart Attack

If a person has a heart attack, the doctors should be called immediately. However, before the medical experts come, Reiki can be administered to the upper and lower abdomen. Remember that the energy of the universe should not be given directly to the heart.

First Position

Place one hand on the right side of the lowest ribs while the other hand goes underneath it.

Second Position

One hand should be placed above the navel and the other hand below it.

Third Position

The healer's hand should go between the shoulders and shoulder blades.

Fourth Position

The hands should be placed on the lower ribs, above the kidneys.

For general heart trouble, consult a physician before taking any other form of healing.

Epileptic Fits and Weight Problem

Epileptic Fits

For epileptic fits, the universal energy should flow into the spine between the shoulder blades. The sessions should only take place before or after a seizure.

First Position

The healer's hand should cup the back of the recipient's head with his or her fingertips placed on the medulla oblongata.

Second Position

The hands should cover the front section of the neck, avoiding making contact with it.

Third Position

One hand has to stay above the navel with the other hand below it.

Weight Problem

First Position

From the forehead region of the top teeth, the practitioner should place his or her hands in a parallel position to the left and right of the nose.

Second Position

The hands should cover the front section of the neck without touching it so that the recipient feels comfortable.

Third Position

Place one hand above the navel, while the other hand goes below it.

Fourth Position

Use the ball of the thumbs on the ridges of the pelvic bones with the tips of the hands close to each other at the pubic bone, forming a V.

Fifth Position

Place the hands on the shoulder blades.

Sixth Position

One hand has to be placed across the sacral plate while the other one stays vertically below with a little bit more pressure.

Seventh Position

The hands are placed around the ankles.

Anemia

Anemia can be taken care of with the universal energy channeled at the top of the head using the positions below.

First Position

With the hands cupping the back of the head, the fingertips should be placed on the medulla oblongata.

Second Position

One hand should be placed on the lowest ribs on the right side, while the other is underneath it.

Third Position

Place your hands on the left lower rib and then below it.

Cancer and Fever

For cancer, it is crucial to perform regular treatment for the entire body while channeling the hand positions that you will find below with universal energy.

First Position

With one hand on the lowest ribs on the right side, the other hand can be placed below it.

Second Position

One hand should be placed above the navel and the other hand goes below it.

Third Position

The practitioner should place one hand across the thymus while the other is at the right angle below and between the breasts, forming a T. The total duration for this position should be between 15 to 20 minutes.

There can be cases in which the cancer patient is extremely weak. In this situation, it is vital to balance the chakras. The hand positions below will be helpful.

For Frail Recipients

First Position

One hand should be placed across the sacral plate and the other hand goes vertically below it with no pressure.

Second Position

The hands are placed at the soles of the feet with the big toes covered from the tips.

Tongue Cancer

For tongue cancer, Reiki has to be channeled in the body from the feet. If it is breast or urogenital cancer, it matters to do intensive Reiki at the second chakra with particular attention paid to the hand positions below.

First Position

The balls of the thumb should be on the ridges of the pelvis while the tips of the hands should be placed close to each other at the pubic bone, forming a V.

Second Position

One hand is placed across the sacral plate with the other hand goes vertically below with no pressure.

Third Position

The hands are placed around the ankles.

Leukemia

For leukemia, Reiki treatment should be used for the whole body, and the recommended positions below are excellent.

First Position

The healer should place one hand on the lowest ribs on the right side while the other hand is directly underneath it.

Second Position

The hands should be placed on the lower left ribs and then below it.

Third Position

The balls of the thumb should be placed on the ridges of the pelvic bones while the tips of the hands should be close to each other at the pubic bone, forming a V.

Fourth Position

With one hand placed across the sacral plate, the other hand should be placed vertically below it with no pressure.

Fifth Position

The practitioner's hands should be placed around the ankles.

Sixth Position

The hands should be placed on the soles of the feet with the big toes covered from the tips.

Fever

First Position

From the forehead region of the top teeth, the practitioner should place his or her hands in a parallel position to the right and left of the nose.

Second Position

The hands should be placed on the recipient's ears.

Third Position

The hands should be covering the front section of the neck without touching it.

Fourth Position

Place the hands on the left lower ribs and below it.

Fifth Position

Place one hand across the thymus and the other hand at a right angle position below and between the breasts. Let both hands form a T. Now, there can be a temporary surge of temperature when this is applied, but it will be followed swiftly by great relief.

Cramps and Leg Problems

Cramps

Cramps can be very discomforting, and the most common ones take place in the leg area. Hence, this section will present the hand positions that you can use to achieve Reiki treatment for and leg problems.

First Position

The hands should be placed in a parallel manner from the forehead to the region of the top teeth and then right and left of the nose.

Second Position

The healer's hands should be on the lowest ribs on the right side and then below it.

Third Position

The hands are placed on the shoulder blades.

Fourth Position

Place the hands on the lower ribs, above the kidney.

Fifth Position

The hands should cover the hollows of the knee.

Sixth Position

The hands should be placed on the soles of the feet with the big toes covered from the tips.

Leg Problems

First Position

Hands should be placed from the forehead region of the top teeth and to the parallel position of the right and left sides of the nose.

Second Position

One hand should be across the sacral plate, while the other hand is placed vertically below with no pressure.

Third Position

The hands should cover the hollows of the recipient's knee.

Fourth Position

For the fourth position, the hands should be placed around the ankles.

Fifth Position

Place the hands on the soles of the feet with the big toes covered from the tips.

Blood Pressure and Bleeding

The positions you will find below will aid the Reiki treatment for bleeding, as well as high or low blood pressure.

Bleeding

If you notice that the bleeding is severe and consistent, then you will need to administer first aid. However, for small bleedings, Reiki can be used to heal the wound.

First Position

The healer should place his or her hands from the forehead to the region of the upper teeth in a parallel position from the right to left nose.

Second Position

The hands should cover the front section of the neck to pass on universal energy without touching the neck.

Third Position

The practitioner's hands should be on the lower side of the left ribs and below it.

Fourth Position

The hands are to be placed on the lower ribs, above the kidney.

Fifth Position

The hands should cover the hollows of the knee.

High Blood Pressure

First Position

The hands should be placed on the front section of the neck. As always, try not to apply too much pressure or touch the neck.

Second Position

Place the hands on the lower side of the left ribs and below it.

Third Position

The hands should be at the soles of the feet with the big toes covered from the tips.

Low Blood Pressure

First Position

The practitioner's hands are to be placed between the shoulders and shoulder blades.

Second Position

Move the hands on the shoulder blades. Hold this position for a while.

Third Position

With one hand on the sacral plate, the other hand can be placed vertically below it with more pressure.

Fourth Position

Place the hands on the soles of the feet, and the big toes should be covered from the tips.

Detoxification

The Reiki treatment for detoxification requires sessions for the entire body until signs of healing start to show forth. Some of them include darker urine with a different smell, better bowel movements, and sweating. The recipient should also have a regular intake of water, lots of rest periods, and showers.

If you are experiencing challenges with your liver, then you need to consult a physician for proper medical checks.

First Position

The healer should place his or her hands from the forehead to the region of the top teeth in a parallel position, moving to the right and left of the nose.

Second Position

This position should be done on the neck, and it works directly on thyroid and parathyroid gland, as well as on the larynx, vocal cords, and lymph nodes.

Third Position

Place one hand on the lowest ribs on the right side. Put the other hand below it, too.

Fourth Position

One hand should be placed on the lower side of the left ribs and below it.

Fifth Position

Place one hand on the navel and the other below it.

Sixth Position

One hand should be placed across the thymus while the other is at a right angle below and between the breasts, forming a T.

Seventh Position

The balls of the thumb should be placed on the ridges of the pelvic bones with the tips of the hands close to each other at the pubic bone, forming a V.

Eight Position

The hands should be placed on the lower ribs, above the kidney.

Ninth Position

With one hand placed across the sacral plate, the other hand should be vertically below it with more pressure.

Tenth Position

The hands should be placed on the soles of the feet, and the big toes should be covered from the tips.

Bladder Problems and Acne

Bladder Problems

These positions will work well with you if you experience severe bladder problems.

First Position

The practitioner should cup the back of the recipient's head with the fingertips placed on the medulla oblongata.

Second Position

The balls of the thumb are placed on the ridges of the pelvic bones with the tips of the hands close to each other at the pubic bone, forming a V.

Third Position

Place the hands between the shoulders and the shoulder blades.

Fourth Position

One hand goes across the sacral plate, and the other is placed below it vertically with increased pressure.

Fifth Position

The hands should be placed around the knees.

Acne

For acne, the Reiki treatment should begin with the whole body for a few days. Then, the following sessions should be done with more focus on the affected area.

First Position

The hands should cover the neck (front section) while being careful to avoid causing any discomfort to the recipient.

Second Position

The hands are placed on the lower ribs, above the kidney.

Third Position

The practitioner should place one hand on the lowest ribs on the right side and the other hand underneath it.

Fourth Position

Next, one hand is placed on the navel and the other below it.

Fifth Position

For the last position, the balls of the thumb should be placed on the ridges of the pelvic bones with the tips of the hands close to each other at the pubic bone, forming a V.

Rheumatism

First Position

One hand should be placed above the navel with the other below it.

Second Position

The balls of the thumb should be placed on the ridges of the pelvic bones with the tips of the hands close to each other at the pubic bone, forming a V.

Third Position

The hands are to be placed on the lower ribs, above the kidney.

Fourth Position

The hands should cover the hollows of the knee.

Menstrual Complaints and Childbirth

First Position

One hand should be on the lowest ribs on the right side with the other directly below it.

Second Position

One hand is placed above the navel and the other goes below it.

Third Position

The balls of the thumb should be placed on the ridges of the pelvic bones with the tips of the hands close to each other at the pubic bone, forming a V.

Fourth Position

The hands should be placed on the shoulder blades.

Fifth Position

With one hand across the sacral plate, the other hand should be placed below in a vertical position with a bit more pressure.

Sixth Position

The hands should be placed around the ankles.

Seventh Position

The hands should be placed on the soles of the feet, and the big toes should be covered from the tips.

Childbirth

Reiki can help expectant mothers enjoy a relaxing experience that makes the process of childbirth easier. It also aids the opening of the pelvis, which makes the delivery less painful. However, the following hand positions must be used before the D-day.

First Position

One hand should be placed above the navel and the other below it.

Second Position

The healer should place the balls of the thumb on the pelvic bones with the tips close to each other at the pubic bone, forming a V.

Third Position

The hands should be placed on the lower ribs, above the kidney.

Fourth Position

One hand should be placed across the sacral plate, which is the bone plate above the fold of the buttocks. The other hand should be placed below it vertically with a little bit of pressure for easy contact with universal energy.

Nose Complaints

In addition to the hand positions that you will utilize for this ailment, you should also use local treatment. The ones you will find below are for three forms of noise-related health challenges that cut across nosebleeds, sinus problems, and nose blockages.

Nose Blockage

First Position

A healer should place hands in a parallel position to the right and left of the nose from the forehead to the region of the top teeth.

Second Position

One hand should be placed on the lowest ribs on the right side, with the other hand directly below.

Third Position

With one hand placed across the thymus, the other hand should be at a right angle below and between the breasts, forming a T.

Sinus Problem

For sinus problems, use the positions above, along with the ones you will find below.

First Position

The balls of the thumb should be placed on the pelvic ridges with the tips of the hands close to each other at the pubic bone, forming a V.

Second Position

The hands should then be placed on the shoulder blades.

Third Position

One hand should be placed across the sacral plate which is the bone plate just above the folds of the buttocks and the other hand placed in a vertical position below. This time, however, there should be a little more pressure.

Fourth Position

The hands should be placed around the ankles.

Nosebleed

First Position

The hands should cup the back of the head with fingertips placed on the medulla oblongata. Ensure that your fingertips are on the soft spot that you can feel when they are passed along the midline of the head to the neck. This should be where half the hard bone ends (that's how you locate the medulla oblongata).

Second Position

The hands should cover the front section of the neck. With this position, the universal energy will lead to the nasal organ as the nose is firmly connected to the throat.

Third Position

One hand should be placed above the navel and the other hand below it.

Fourth Position

The hands should be placed between the shoulders and shoulder blades.

Fifth Position

Finally, place the hands alone on the shoulder blades and release the universal energy.

Cold, Cough, Insomnia, and Allergies

Common cold can lead to several other issues if left unchecked. When you have insomnia, after all, there is a higher possibility of various diseases settling in your body because you don't get good sleep, which is a requirement for a healthy and robust body. Allergies can also be very discomforting. However, with the right Reiki hand positions, you can get a cure for all three issues.

Cold

First Position

The healer should place his or her hands from the forehead to the areas around the top teeth and the left side of the nose.

Second Position

The hands should cover the front section of the neck, but the healer should avoid touching the neck directly as it can lead to discomfort and fear in some people.

Third Position

One hand should be placed across the thymus and the other hand at the right angle below and between the breasts, forming a T. This position channels the Reiki's healing energy into the recipient's body with each hand movement.

Insomnia

For insomnia, channeling Reiki to the collarbone is highly effective.

First Position

The hands should be placed in a parallel position to the right and left side of the nose from the forehead to the region of the top teeth.

Second Position

Place the hands on the temples with fingertips getting to the cheekbones.

Third Position

One hand should be placed above the navel and the other one below it.

Fourth Position

The balls of the practitioner's thumb should be placed on the ridges of the pelvic bones, and the tips of the hands should be close to each other at the pubic bone, forming a V.

Allergies

Whole-body treatment is usually the beginning of a Reiki treatment for allergies, with a focus on the specific regions where the reactions manifest.

First Position

The hands should cover the front section of the neck, but do not touch the neck.

Second Position

The hands should be placed in a parallel position to the left and right sides of the nose from the forehead to the top teeth region.

Third Position

The balls of the thumb should be placed on the ridges of the pelvic bones with the tips of the hands close to each other at the pubic bone, creating a V.

Fourth Position

One hand should be placed above the navel and the other hand below it.

Give the recipient a few minutes to rest after each session and monitor health progress closely to decide on a continuance with sessions and the duration for the meetings.

When we say that the world is beginning to adopt the Reiki approach for treatment, the content of this chapter has provided insight into the reasons for their interest. Reiki truly has immense potential. The more you learn about its abilities, the more exciting it gets because there are layers to unravel with every session. Not to mention, it gets better with time.

Nevertheless, there are also additional benefits to using Reiki for treatment purposes. We just concentrated on the aspect of illnesses and diseases in this chapter. In the next chapter, we will take you through the other perks that will touch your mind, as well as your emotional balance.

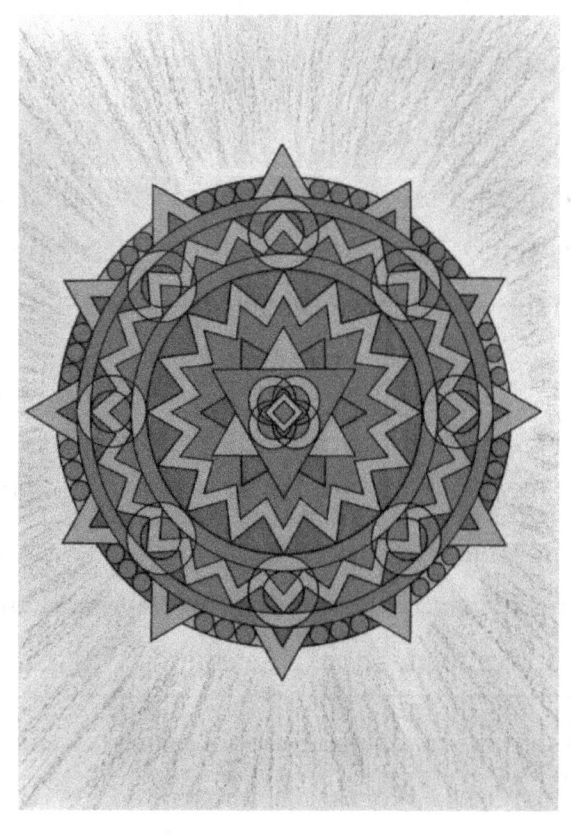

Chapter Five: Additional Benefits of Reiki

Isn't it amazing that we have probably embarked on this journey with you knowing little or nothing about Reiki, and now you know not only what it is about but also how to administer it as a practitioner and receive it as a recipient?

The journey with this book only validates the fact that there is so much to unearth about Reiki. The more you learn, the more you want to discover about it. We have built solid foundations that have created an enabling environment for understanding all things, but we are ready to take things up a notch.

Most of the information you will find everywhere else about Reiki focuses solely on the health benefits that individuals can enjoy. By saying 'health' here, we are referring to physical relief from illnesses and diseases.

However, there is so much more to Reiki than that. Of course, it is essential that we seek such help, but wouldn't it be great if we expand our knowledge about it?

When we started, I told you that this is a comprehensive book that doesn't just cover the basics of the subject matter but also goes deeper to present information about Reiki. Hence, in this chapter, we are going to consider its other benefits that don't focus on illnesses alone.

Through this chapter, you will realize that Reiki is a treatment option that offers so much more to you with a few sessions. The perks that you will find here are not similar to the ones that we have discussed in the previous section. They do not come with hand positions either.

You will get to learn another approach to weighing in on the benefits that Reiki provides. You will also realize that the treatment goes beyond what happens to your body and cuts across what occurs inside it, as well as in your mind.

Additional Psychological and Mental Benefits of Reiki

Accelerates Self-Healing Ability

Reiki healing makes it easier for your body to return to its natural state of being able to heal itself from within. This is made possible by the life force energy associated with Reiki.

Your body starts to move in the right direction as your breathing, heart rate, and blood pressure improves. When you self-treat with Reiki or get healing from someone else, one of the first activities that you will do during every session is to breathe deeply. When you practice and perfect deep breathing, your mind will get settled naturally.

As your respiration gets stronger, your body opens up to receive new energy and expels the negative one. The process of being able to do so can accelerate your body's self-healing abilities as it is a correctional process with long-term mental and psychological benefits.

The body was created to self-heal, but it started to lose its natural touch when we exposed our mind and thought processes to contradictory ideas. So, for you to return to that natural state of self-healing, you must introduce something from the universe again. This is where Reiki becomes very powerful.

The more universal energy you are exposed to, the more you can strike a balance with your natural self-healing state. So, instead of you falling ill all the time, you may stronger, optimistic about life, and energized to do more.

Gets Rid of Bad Karma

Bad karma is likened to a blockage in your system. Now, when your artery is blocked, the blood flow to your heart is reduced, and it may lead to a cardiac arrest. This explanation with blood flow perfectly captures the situation that goes on in your life when you have bad karma around you. You start to feel like your energy and will to live a better life is trapped. With the manifestation of adverse events, you tend to believe that life is unfair.

You will also believe that the reason why other people seem to have a more comfortable life is that the universe favors them more than you. Get rid of lousy karma using the universal energy and avoid getting trapped energy. After all, the latter manifests through depression, irritability, and other forms of physical problems.

Reiki helps in cleansing your karma, and the blockages can be removed by a Reiki master as he or she can channel the energy of the universe through themselves into your body to cleanse the bad karma surrounding you.

When bad karma is taken care of, you will feel that the energy around you is better and that you have been empowered to live your life to its fullest potential. If you keep up with the Reiki sessions, then you will get rid of it forever!

Improves Quality of Life

When we talk about the quality of life, we do not only refer to how you live in terms of the material things, e.g., your home, cars, clothes, etc. We are more focused on the quality of your daily experiences. What you go through every day eventually sums up the kind of life you are generally living.

If most of your days are challenge-ridden, you can easily overcome so many issues that leave you feeling less motivated in the long run. Then, there is a problem somewhere. It means that there are negative energies that have crept into your consciousness and are making it difficult for you to embrace the good stuff in your life.

With universal energy, not only can you embrace the good things you have going for yourself, but you also get to become aware of them and intentionally focus on it instead of being worried about what isn't working.

There will be things that you will surely have to deal with, such as personal challenges, but you don't need to make these things the center of your existence. Allow the quality of your life get an improvement with universal energy; let your chakras and bodily energies become aligned towards one goal, which is being the best version of yourself and living your best life today.

After Reiki sessions, you will realize that the good things you can do to add some quality into your life aren't so tricky at all. Concentrate on the little things, smile a lot, and seek happiness from within. All of this can be made possible with consistent exposure to the universal energy.

Improves Sleep

A significant outcome when you receive Reiki is relaxation, which aids you in getting better sleep. We become strong enough to combat fatigue and other illnesses attributed to a lack of quality sleep this way.

We mentioned earlier that some Reiki recipients fall asleep during sessions, but it doesn't end with the Reiki meetings. A few of them continue that way after the sessions because they have received a renewed energy that keeps them at peace with themselves.

The thoughts and issues that keep you awake at night enough not to get good sleep can be taken care of with universal energy. One of the significant aims of Reiki is to empower you with the inner energy that your body requires for self-care.

So, you wouldn't need to actively do a lot of things on your own as there is an energy force within you now that causes everything else about your life to align correctly, even your sleep patterns. If you have been struggling with getting the recommended hours of sleep or you have discovered that you cannot stay in bed throughout the night, then you need Reiki sessions.

If you think that by doing nothing about this sleep deprivation challenge you are helping yourself as you hope, you need to rethink your actions. Why do you think people take sleeping pills? When you have a sleep issue, you don't sit and wait it out. Instead, you do something!

In this case, you wouldn't have to take pills or resort to other forms of drugs that you may have to enjoy the Reiki process and bask in the feel of it while getting better sleep subsequently.

Promotes Spiritual Growth and Emotional Cleansing

People erroneously believe that they need to be into spirituality before they can enjoy the benefits of Reiki, and this isn't true. You don't need to be an enthusiastic, spiritual being before taking in the universal energy.

When you experience spiritual growth, you will notice that it does so much more for your mind as you will feel at peace with yourself more and be contented with life. Reiki doesn't only address specific issues; it also focuses on the whole person. So, when you go for sessions, feeling less wholesome spiritually, you can be sure of experiencing a subtle shift from deep within your being.

Suddenly you have guidance on what to do, you are inspired to make attitudinal changes for the better, and your take on situations are better framed from a fresh perspective instead of the normal thought processes you imbibed in the past.

Listen, sometimes you don't need a lot of people giving you advice, what you need is to have an improved inner conviction that helps you make decisions and stand boldly with the choice you made because you know you did the correct thing.

So now, other people can come to you for emotional advice as well because you have gotten your life together and you are leaning more on the spiritual energy acquired from Reiki instead of your intuition. Emotional cleansing makes it possible for you to overlook the wrongs of those who hurt you and move on gracefully because you know your life isn't defined by how you feel about others.

A lot of people who complain about some fundamental mental issues need to experience emotional cleansing, and they will be fine. Let the universal energy protect your mind from adverse emotional reactions and help you see beyond the pain or hurt you may feel.

Speeds Up Recovery From Illnesses and Surgeries

If you discover that it always takes you a long time to recover from diseases and operations, then you will need universal energy. Reiki speeds up recovery from illnesses and surgeries as the periods after treatment can be a very complicated one that, if not properly managed, may cause the individual to experience a relapse.

For some people, the reason why they are unable to recover swiftly may be because of the side effects of drugs and surgical procedures. However, Reiki can help them adjust to the medicine or treatment that they are given by reducing the impact of side effects.

If you have had surgery recently, wait for a few days and then take on a Reiki session to solidify the healing process. You may not have to take on more than one session because you are also taking drugs or other forms of medicine. After the first one, though, discuss your feelings with the healer so that he or she can ascertain if you will need more sessions.

After a medical treatment, your body may still be trying to normalize again, which means that it needs support. To be specific, it needs a life force energy that can enhance the impact of the treatment that you have received.

After your Reiki session, you will notice that whatever pain you felt after surgery or treatment is gone or has subsided, it is mainly because of the impact of universal energy. The same way Reiki helps new mothers after delivery gets better is how it helps others regain their health and vitality.

You don't need more drugs to take care of your post-surgery or post-treatment period. What you need is an energy force field that moves through your body, recreating a stronger response to the medical procedures you have gone through.

Guarantees Mental Freedom

A lot of people are physically free, but they are not mentally free. Hence, they deal with an inner self-identity struggle that sets them in a prison of the mind. "I feel free" is often the statement made by Reiki recipients after their sessions. Some individuals may not even be able to describe this feeling aptly, but they know that something was taken away, and something more powerful released inside them.

The concept of mental freedom isn't discussed well enough because some people do not even know it exists. They are not familiar with the idea; that's why they don't know when they are mentally free and when they are not. The inability to make your own decisions and seek the validation of others makes you feel mentally caged.

Reiki can help you regain freedom through exciting sessions that make it possible for you to feel empowered and comfortable with yourself enough to trust your decisions. A person who is mentally free doesn't need to prove anything to anyone.

In the social media-inspired world we live in today, if a person can stay true to themselves, that individual will surely do exploits and be known as a leader in any field of endeavor.

If you want to know if you are mentally free, check your decisions and the impact that other people have over your mind. Then, if you are not satisfied with your findings, take on Reiki. After the session, you will testify to the fact that there is something known as mental freedom.

Don't shut your mind off from the help it needs; let Reiki step in and make a difference. As you learn to rely on Reiki for these small things, you will learn how to trust the process when dealing with huge issues entirely.

The state of your mind determines the state of your life, so choose freedom today by sticking to the universal energy for a reformed mental state. Whatever you do will always be a reflection of your mental freedom or otherwise. With Reiki, you have an opportunity to experience mental freedom for a long time.

Assists the Body in Eliminating Toxins

Reiki plays a very active role in supporting the body's immune system by cleaning out toxins. Through Reiki, our bodies are reminded to shift into the parasympathetic nervous system's self-healing mode.

Resting doesn't mean that you have to stop working or doing the things you love. It just means that your body will be signaled to sleep and digest better, which is crucial for the maintenance of health and vitality. The more time you spend in the Reiki space, the more active and productive you will be without feeling stressed out, having burn-outs, or getting exhausted.

If there are toxins in your body that builds up gradually, there is a higher chance that you wouldn't know until it becomes too late and you break down with an ailment. So, Reiki spots those toxins and helps it get rid of them before they constitute a bigger problem for you.

With toxins gone, your body will not experience imbalances anymore, and you can rest easy knowing that a major cause of illness has been defeated.

Promotes Natural Balance Between Mind, Body, and Spirit

A significant reason why you go through some days feeling less accomplished even though you put in so much effort is that there is a lack of harmony between the three most important aspects of your life, such as your body, mind, and spirit.

Sometimes your mind tells you to do something, and you find yourself doing something else, which leads to unrest within your spirit. With regular Reiki treatment, you can achieve greater harmony with these three elements such that you also strike a natural between them.

Mental balance enhances learning, mental clarity, and memory. It helps an individual cope with stress and alleviates mood swings. When your energies are correctly positioned, you will find that there are no confusions in your life.

All your decisions (mental, physical, and spiritual) will be in sync because they are all in alignment. This also means that your relationships will be purposeful, and you will be able to deal wisely with everyone else. We should all strive for balance in life. However, more importantly, we should aim to attain it in the long run.

Reiki helps you achieve balance and enables you to stick to it by empowering your mind to always to be attuned with your spirit and your body. This way, you wouldn't feel like you are doing anything contradictory the next time you make a decision. Your life will be like a natural flowing stream with no waves and complete calm as events unfold.

With Reiki, you can also stay centered in the present moment instead of getting caught up in the regrets and mistakes of the past. You will even notice if you have a harmonious reaction to people. For example, it is possible that in the past you told someone that you accept their apology, but in your mind, you are still upset about what they did.

When you use Reiki long enough, as you tell the person you have accepted his or her apology, it will be the same thing in your mind and spirit. There will be no grudges or hidden bitterness, thus helping you become a better person.

Reduces Depression and Anxiety

Reiki is very instrumental in aiding changes with your mood. The root causes of depression and anxiety are negative moods that rub off on everything else about you. With Reiki, you tend to feel better and more positive because you are receiving life force energy that dissolves energetic blockages.

It is difficult for a person who is continuously exposed to life force energy to become depressed or anxious. Once you come in contact with this energy form, your life gets better. No one is saying that you wouldn't have challenges, but even with them, you will be able to overcome them, thus avoiding being depressed or anxious.

In addition to a significant reduction with anxious and depressed feelings, you will also observe that you no longer give room for anger in your life. All of them (depression, violence, and anxiety) are negative expressions of being dissatisfied with life.

However, with Reiki, there are no negativities, which means that universal energy is the best form of treatment that you need to fight off depression and anxiety. Reiki works by helping you boost your mood because, when you have improved moods, anxiety tends to wear out, and you look at the world with the eyes of positivity.

Depression leads to a loss of vigor and excitement to do the things that you love, but you can regain all of that after a Reiki session(s). Remember that Reiki permeates all aspects of your body and its general composition, including the material and non-material ones.

So, when you go for Reiki session, you should tell the healer that you are dealing with depression and get it out of your system for good. However, what happens after the session? What if I start to feel anxious afterwards? There are fewer chances of you going back to that path again after getting healed because the meeting balances your chakra and resets the root causes of the problem in your mind.

Do not think about getting depressed again. Focus on enjoying your new mental freedom, and you will be able to sustain it. We will discuss sustainability in the next chapter, so look out for that section.

Eases Pain

There are several reasons for pain in the body, but one thing we can all agree on is the fact that it isn't pleasant. From shoulder to wrist pain, back pain, etc. working hours, age, and sleeping or sitting positions can be responsible for pain in the body.

While you are advised to make corrections with some of these cases, you can use universal energy to reverse the impact of the pain in your body. Reiki is about motion. The energy is always in motion, while pain represents something that is stuck somewhere in the body.

So, when universal energy sets in, it flows through your body and gets those stuck energies and blockages out, thus causing immediate or gradual relief to your body. However, listen to this, if you go back to the activities and things that cause you to feel the pain, you will be creating a vicious circle for yourself. The Reiki healer will probably tell you this, too.

Get your healing and go back to the office to make changes on the chair that isn't good for your back, join a gym, or become active with exercises that will keep pain at bay. Yes, Reiki can help, but you have to do better with things you can avoid. Once you use Reiki to take care of yourself with regards pain, make sure that your health is your priority, and you are proactive with maintaining the results that you have gotten with Reiki.

Reduces Stress

Stress reduction is one of the most popular benefits of Reiki. Even if you have booked a session for something else, one thing is for sure: you would come back feeling less stressed out in addition to the benefits you booked the session for.

Most sicknesses and diseases today are linked to stress. There's environmental anxiety, emotional stress, work-related stress, or even self-induced stress. All of these patterns will lead to irregular heartbeat, eating disorders, mood swings, and even sexual problems.

So, most of the time, a person carries the weight of being stressed on his or her shoulders. However, when they show up for a Reiki session, and the healer places his or her hands on their shoulders, they can feel the stress slowly ebb away.

Universal energy can trigger a more satisfying feeling within you that makes it possible for you to concentrate on what you can do instead of taking on too much at a time. More importantly, you will intentionally stay off anything that will induce stress after the Reiki session because your body has gotten a glimpse into how life can be without feeling stressed all the time.

Universal energy has the potential to help you redefine your life and become a protector of your mind space, in the sense that the decisions you make are not solely influenced by what you can do for others (which puts you under a lot of pressure) but based on what you can satisfactorily and with peace of mind.

It is safe to say that aside from the benefits you get from Reiki sessions, you are also passively taught how to treat yourself and make better decisions. You are encouraged to take care of your mental space because, if anything goes wrong in there, something can go wrong anywhere else.

Heals Infection and Inflammation

There are some treatments or surgeries that a person goes through that leads to inflammation in the body or infection without the person even realizing it. Some people will say that they feel weak with abnormal body temperature. They try to get treated for it without realizing that it is the fault of the inflammation or infection.

If you had surgery recently or just got cured of a disease or ailment, pay attention to how you feel for the next couple of days.

If you don't feel great even after taking drugs, try Reiki.

Sometimes the healing that comes from Reiki when dealing with inflammation or infection may seem like a miracle because it is often instant. You can live an infection free life every day. It isn't an assumption but a possibility. Still, first, you know what to do and stick to it.

Reiki isn't just an option for ailments. When inflammation and infections are not well taken care of, then it can lead to severe illnesses. So, using Reiki against the disease shouldn't be done after a health scare but as a preventive measure to keep the body in check at all times.

When Reiki therapy is administered, you will find that you are relieved of the anxiety and worry that these issues may have caused you. The more focused you are on getting more universal energy, the more your body builds the resistance against inflammation and infection.

When we say Reiki helps you maintain good health or keeps you healthy, this is an example of how it works because a person who is free from infection and inflammation long-term is on the path to sustainable health.

Helps You Feel Empowered

The reason a lot of people struggle with the feeling of empowerment is that they are never calm enough to get to know who they are and accept themselves that way. The busier they are, the more distant they become, and this makes them feel empowered.

Reiki has a potent and calming effect. You will always feel calm in your sessions, and when you are in that calm state, you experience the freedom to accept your flaws and embrace the good qualities you embody.

This also means you become aware of the character traits you need to work on. As you work on them, you feel empowered because, unlike in the past, no one can use these flaws against you anymore. Hopelessness also goes away when universal energy is introduced. A recipient once said that after the session, he felt like a brand-new man, and this is the reason why he feels empowered as well.

Empowerment gives you the ability to take charge of your life by steering it in the direction that you want. To be more explicit, the power will be in your hands. With everything you've learned thus far, you know that the hands are very potent with universal energy.

Even when you are not in a Reiki session with a healer, you can practice it on yourself to create a lasting impact. You can always rely on it whenever you feel less empowered. Take advantage of the calming effect that Reiki offers by being fully immersed in every session so that there can be a deep fellowship with yourself and the universal energy.

So many things can be corrected in your life when you feel empowered and not defeated. Reiki is the way to go in bringing that feeling of empowerment to your consciousness.

Increases Creative Juices

If you have always struggled with being innovative, it isn't because you were born that way but because you are consciously or unconsciously blocking off the creative energy. A significant thing that happens in people's lives and is responsible for the lack of creative juices is stress.

Reiki can help you reduce or completely eradicate your stress levels while aiding clarity and focus. When you have not stressed out anymore, and your mind is to streamline to capture new ideas, then you can say your creative juices are back.

Reiki breaks down energetic blocks, and once you are free of these blocks, you tend to find new avenues and inspiration to generate ideas using your imaginative ability. The truth is that the ability has always been there; you didn't acknowledge it because you weren't even conscious of it in the first place.

After a Reiki session, go back to those things you found too difficult to do. Go back to those tasks you needed ideas on and try to get them done. You will observe that there are no more mental restrictions or difficulties because whatever was constituting a mental blockage has been taken care of by Reiki.

Remember that we have mentioned that universal energy does so much more than it's intended for in a given session because it is energy that flows through your body and fixes whatever needs to be fixed. If your challenge is with the creative juices that you need for your job, business, or family, then you can rest easy knowing that universal energy will take care of it for you.

Now, don't try to force the creative juices after a Reiki session. Relax and let it flow; don't doubt or wonder if it will happen because thoughts like that can affect you negatively.

Helps You Magnetize Abundance

Have you ever heard the statement, "You are a product of what you think about the most"? If you had, and you think back to the events in your life, then you will agree that the things you give so much attention to through your thoughts will often manifest. The universe uses a very fair method to present what you desire through your will. If you think you deserve to be happy, then happiness is what you get from the universe.

The same principle applies to everything else in life, from prosperity to abundance. Everything good you desire can come to you just by channeling the right energy, and Reiki is the conduit that you need to tap into to gain the universe's positive energy.

When you show up for a Reiki session, you do not only get to feel the hands of the healed but also learn how to be much more affirmative by using the energy generated through Reiki to touch the things around you. You can see an energy-charged ball transform whatever you want and make it suit your life entirely.

The more you are in contact with the vibration that brings more abundance to people's lives, the more you can attract it into your life. This is why consistent Reiki sessions are always advised. Now, no one is saying that you should show up at the healer's place every day or demand distant healing daily.

You can schedule the sessions to be just about the right amount of time you will need to get the energy for abundance and then magnetize it through self-Reiki sessions.

Creating a comprehensive book like this one takes a lot of effort because of the amount of research required, and we have genuinely achieved so much with the chapters and sections thus far. It is time to wrap up the journey on a very inspiring note.

The next chapter will take you through the process of sustainability with all things Reiki. It will be the last chapter, an opportunity to inspire you to take action so that these benefits can become a palpable experience.

Chapter Six: The Concept of Continuity with Reiki

Do you know why Christmas is always a magical experience for kids? It is because of the continuing tradition with Christmas gifts, Santa Clause, holiday cheer, and every other thing that makes the season special. So, a child goes through this process from a tender age till he or she becomes a teenager and will always remember the magic of Christmas.

Now, Reiki isn't a seasonal experience like Christmas, but it can completely transform your life in a wholesome way. So, why not think about sustaining this feeling?

Some people discover the excitement of Reiki, bask in the feeling for a few days, and forget about the experience. Others, however, do not forget intentionally but say, "Life happens." This is why they must take an intentional approach towards ensuring that they sustain and continue the healing process.

More often than not, when there is a discourse on universal energy and treatment options, there is very little attention to how people can sustain what they learn and keep up with their sessions.

Nothing good will last long if there is no effort to ensure its continuity. You want to make sure that this fantastic experience you have going for yourself continues and that you are inspired to do more with Reiki other than simply know how it works.

This chapter will introduce you to some ideas that will ensure the continuity of your Reiki experience. It is the perfect way to bring this journey to an end.

Note: The steps you will find below cut across what both healers and recipients can do to sustain the practice. So, depending on what you are going after, there is an idea for both sides of the treatment option.

How to Sustain Reiki in Your life

Show Up for Sessions

If you are very serious about sustainability with your Reiki practice and healing, then you must develop the discipline to show up for all your recommended meetings. There is a small group of people who believe that Reiki doesn't work and that it isn't as effective as the healers make it be. Such people speak from the incompetent experiences they had and will do whatever they can to make others believe them.

Well, the reason why they say that is because they didn't complete their sessions or stick to the advice or caution of the practitioners. While others have amazing Reiki stories to tell, they don't. If you don't show up for sessions, you will end up like such person.

It takes a lot of commitment to get the best out of Reiki. In some situations, one session is enough. For others, though, you will need more than one. Still, the decision isn't yours to make, especially if you aren't doing self-treatment. The healer will decide on that because he or she is the one who is handling the session and will know what you need.

If you aspire to become a professional healer someday, how do you intend to help your patients get better when you can't adhere to your own healer's advice? Reiki is never about convenience or a perfectly suited time or when you feel like doing it.

If you have a pressing challenge, and you are keen on taking care of it, you must be willing to do whatever is required to make it happen. We are not talking about achieving healing today and struggling with the same thing the next week; we are seeking ways through which you can become a walking testimony of the impact of Reiki and achieve that. Therefore, consistency with sessions is required.

Now I know that some individuals may have hectic schedules, even though they genuinely want to complete their sessions. If you are such a person, then you must learn how to prioritize and manage your time well enough so that you can do everything necessary.

Reiki practitioners are not just all about helping you with your ailment or psychological challenge. They are also humane individuals who are trained to understand the value of time.

Instead of procrastinating your sessions or not showing up for them at all, reach out to your healer and explain your peculiar situation.

Let the healer know that you are willing to work around your schedule, but you need help. By doing this, you will be helping yourself as you take on so many things at once, which can lead to stress. Now, you want to ensure that you can sustain the Reiki impact. If you don't know how to manage it with your schedule, speak to your healer.

It wouldn't be nice if, after reading this book, you end up like some people who say that Reiki doesn't work because you didn't commit to the process entirely. We have not only been on a journey together with this book, but you have also invested in your life by purchasing it. So, how do you get the dividends of the investment?

You achieve the latter by being committed to the process and ensuring that you give it your best at all times. You can sustain the Reiki impact. Start by not missing out on sessions, and you will be amazed at the level of progress you make with your experience long-term.

Be Attentive to Your Body

Another step that you can take towards sustaining Reiki is being attentive to your body. Reiki is all about energy, and energy is about awareness. In fact, if you are not someone who is easily attuned or discerning of energy around yourself, you surely cannot get the benefits of Reiki long-term. Meaning, if you are not someone who pays close attention to these things, you will need more practice, and the best way to do that is by listening to your body.

Your body speaks to you all the time. The question is, are you listening? Are you paying attention to the signs and signals that it's sending to you? Some people go for a Reiki session; because they are not attentive to their bodies, though, they don't know what takes place in it. They don't know if they have been healed; they cannot feel the energy permeate their bodies. For this reason, they can never succeed with the idea of sustainability as well.

After ensuring that you have not skipped even one session, you should pay close attention to what your body is trying to say to you. That is the only way you can ascertain the extent of healing you've received and anything else.

Below, you will discover a step that advises you to share your experience with others and help them, but how do you intend sharing with them when you don't know what happened to you? When you are sharing your story with people, and they ask questions regarding the impact of Reiki on your body, what will you say? If you haven't been listening to your body, today is an excellent time to start.

Shut out the noise around you for a few minutes every day. Some people call it meditation, but this time you will seek to listen to your voice. When you shut out everything, wait for a few minutes. With your mind's eye, roam around your body and listen to your heartbeat. Does it seem regular to you? Do you feel tired? Is your body saying something through your new sleep duration?

I am so keen on helping you listen to your body because a lot of ailments and problems that people seek Reiki for are preventable if they have paid attention to their bodies. So, in those moments when you listen, if there is something amiss, share it with your healer or practice Reiki on yourself using the hand movements you've been taught earlier.

Over time, you will find that you don't need to run to the hospital every time there is a little health scare because your body communicates with you, and you listen to it. The universal energy that you get through Reiki will also keep your body stable, so you are always healthy, optimistic, and excited about life.

Learn More

It doesn't matter what you think you already know. There is always more to learn, especially if you want to be a Reiki healer or practitioner for a long while. The most successful therapists do not stop learning. In fact, they intentionally study every day because they realize that nothing will stay the same all year long.

If you don't make attempts to learn and discover more about Reiki, you will become obsolete. Hence, you will no longer be as effective as you used to be. As recipients feel like they are not getting help from you, they will seek other Reiki healers, and you will lose clients.

Building a good reputation as a healer is part of the process. You don't become a reputable one all of a sudden. It takes a lot of work, which lies within your ability to make the sessions work.

Don't stop learning Reiki with this book. Read more materials, listen to successful practitioners, attend seminars and workshops, register for personal coaching lessons, and even do some on-the-job training to know what it's like to work with recipients. If you are committed to the idea of sustainability, then it means you want to practice for a long time. For that to happen, you must be committed to continuing and vigorously learning new procedures.

Think about doctors, lawyers, and people in other professions. It takes them quite a while to become professionals; they go through years of training at varying levels of difficulty as well. You are dealing with the idea that will liberate a lot of individuals from their challenges, and you are attuned to the universe. For this reason, you must take your profession seriously as well.

In the olden days when Reiki just became popular, it wasn't so easy for people who desired to become healers to get further training. Some even had to travel to learn from masters. These days, though, technology has made it easier for anyone who is willing to gain knowledge about Reiki.

Meanwhile, if you don't have money to pay for the more exclusive trainings, you can start with the free ones from blogs. There are also online platforms that are solely dedicated to Reiki training. Before adopting any of the approaches you see virtually, make sure that the website is verified and that you are getting authentic content that suits your desire for success with Reiki.

The more you learn and practice, the better you become, and then you can advance to higher heights with your Reiki practice. You wouldn't learn everything within a specified time frame, so I cannot tell you that it will take one or two years. Several doctors with years of experience still get to learn new facts about their profession every day, after all. If you are keen on being the best in this field, therefore, you must be willing to become aggressive and committed to learning.

Don't Be Selfish

This step is so important, and we cannot bring this book to a close without talking about it. If you are practicing or intend to practice Reiki selfishly with the sole aim of making money, you will be causing a lot of harm to your reputation and the field in general.

Do not practice Reiki just because you want to profit from clients or gain control and prestige. You will have a stubborn time proving your expertise if you do that. Also, Reiki isn't about you, your selfish motives, or what you will derive from it.

Reiki is all about the person who is healed, as well as the role of the healer in connecting the life force energy to the recipient. What's most striking is the fact that you will not be able to establish a thriving practice because you would struggle with gaining access to guidance from the spirit.

If your connection to the universal energy doesn't have a strong spiritual base, then you cannot tap into the universe's energy quickly. A motive is significant since, as a healer, you will be the conduit for the healing the recipient will receive. What kind of channel you want to be, a selfish one who only thinks about themselves? Alternatively, do you want to become a selfless channel?

You must get to know what your motives are before taking the next step towards practicing Reiki. Don't decide on becoming an expert because it seems like a good title or business idea. You must look beyond yourself and what you will gain and continually strive to seek the greater good of all men and women who may cross your path.

If you have read through this book, and you feel that stirring sensation within you to make a difference in the world, then it means that Reiki is for you. When you pursue it, you can be sure of gaining success in this field. On the contrary, if all you see is a business opportunity, I will advise you not to take any step further towards becoming a Reiki practitioner now.

Spread the Word, Help Others

Sustainability will not be possible without the people who want to try out Reiki. So, if you are not concerned about anyone else but yourself, why are you reading this book? It is essential for everyone who wants to practice Reiki, as well as the ones who benefit from it, to take a step forward by reaching out to others.

Think about this for a second. If the earliest practitioners didn't try to help other people, would we ever know about Reiki today? You see, this step has been in use for years now because it is the one thing that guarantees sustainability.

This book and several others in this niche were written by seasoned authors who want to contribute their know-how to the sustainability movement by keeping the topic alive within most human interactions. Hence, if you have a successful Reiki story, why aren't you sharing it?

People only believe what they know can happen. We trust medicines, hospitals, and doctors because we have been taking drugs since we were kids and getting cured of illnesses. However, imagine if a doctor comes forward and says something can work, but he or she doesn't have any proof. Will you believe this physician and take a chance?

Theoretical knowledge doesn't inspire people. After all, anyone can write anything they want. Nevertheless, when individuals hear your distinct story when they know that this thing can transform their lives for good in ways they can only imagine, they will be willing to take a step towards it.

There are two ideas that are related to sustainability. The first one is the concept of spreading the word, and the second one is the concept of helping others. You cannot do one and leave the other. As you take steps towards spreading the word about Reiki, to be specific, you will have to reach out to help others as well.

Now, you don't have to take on an entire neighborhood or a bunch of people at the same time. Sart with your closest friends and family members who may be dealing with one health challenge or another. Introduce them to Reiki and then explain in detail what Reiki is about. If they have questions, try to provide answers but do not exaggerate anything so that they will not have to hold on to unrealistic expectations. If they are keen on books, you can share this book with them.

Considering your loved ones are excited about Reiki enough to want to give it a try, then you can use the second approach, which entails helping others. You try a Reiki treatment session on them to help with their challenge. If you have been self-treating yourself, and you haven't healed someone else before, it may feel strange to you at first. Still, there's no need to worry because we know that you can do this!

Just ensure that you have practiced on yourself long enough and that you have achieved results before helping someone else. Doing self-treatment and treating others are the same. Only, with the latter, you will be channeling the universal energy into someone else's body.

Even if you have a friend who is far away, you can use the distant healing techniques you were taught earlier to make it happen. The point is that, by reaching out to others who need help, you will not only be contributing positively to someone else's life, but you will also be advancing your skills and getting better every day.

Take some time off to practice so that you can feel confident about what you are doing. Sustainability is all about carrying on with the tradition we gained (as others did before us). It is your contribution to the Reiki story. Although it may not be a story that is told globally, in your little way, you will be adding value to the lives of others.

There is more to say and achieve with Reiki, so take time to dig in through research. As you learn more, you will become empowered to share with the world what you have gained. Most healers are inspired by their desire to make the world a better place, to be honest. They see their gift not as a skill but as a medium through which they can contribute positively to the well-being of others.

Experience and Heart (Passion)

If you want to be a successful Reiki practitioner, it is crucial that you become conscious of the concept of experience and heart.

A lot of times, when people discover what they love and what they want to do, they often stick to the books and materials that instruct them how to garner experience. Others take on the job so seriously because they want to be at the top of the game. Well, it is significant to be concerned about the experience, but what about passion?

No one is hugely successful at whatever they do without being passionate about it. For sustainability to become effective with your practice, therefore, there must be room for passion in yourself.

Passion keeps a practitioner going even when it seems like he or she is dealing with daunting challenges.

Make no mistake about this; the experience can never replace passion, regardless of how experienced you are. It is possible that you will throw in the towel and give up sooner than later because you lack passion. Passion is that feeling of excitement you have within you that helps you navigate through the process of helping others with ease.

Some people are highly paid in their jobs, for instance. They have this fantastic office and everything else going for them. However, it turns out that they despise their position. Yes, they enjoy the perks the job brings, but they always think about how different their lives would have been if they could do something they love. Similarly, the bank executive with a cool ride and a driver may be thinking about the passion that he or she has for baking.

Life can be funny like this sometimes. You have an opportunity right now to make this Reiki practice work. This way, you don't end up feeling like you have made a mistake later on. By making it work, I mean building experience and passion at the same time.

First, you become passionate about something by making sure that this is what you want to do. Then, you start practicing it. However, you don't stop working on your passion every day. The best way to keep your determination burning is by going over and beyond everyone else to do the most as a Reiki practitioner.

Show up every day at your workspace with so much glee and excitement like you haven't been doing this for a while, for instance. Don't get too comfortable or too familiar with the process as well. Otherwise, it will become like a regular job. Remember, people are not passionate about regular jobs!

The combination of passion and experience is unbeatable. You will watch yourself rise like an edifice in this field. You will become even more productive with your recipients as there will be a lot of success stories from your sessions. Still, you must provide an answer to the all-important question, "Do I want to be a Reiki healer?"

Don't rush off to answer this one. Take some time to think about it with all the information you have received so far. Try to think objectively without emotional affiliations or any pressure.

Being a Reiki practitioner is excellent but being a passionate one who is poised to garner more experience is exceptionally perfect!

We used a mini portion of this book to discuss the history of Reiki and mentioned some of the individuals in the past who did well with it. Well, those people are still talked about today in Reiki circles because they weren't just experienced but also passionate about what they did to help others. That feeling, combined with experience, made them great in this field. You can enjoy the same process as well if you try to discover what you are passionate about and how you can build your Reiki experience.

When you get a job for the first time in a firm that you love so much, for instance, from your first day at work, you already start to strategize regarding how you are going to get promoted to the top and get a corner office. The reason why you have such ambition is that you don't want to be stagnant in life.

Work With an Illumined Being

Another way through which you can improve your effectiveness with Reiki is by developing a working relationship with an illumined being. Yes, there are Reiki guides who help us with our sessions, but they may not be able to provide you with the highest form of help available. So, you will need to develop a working relationship with an illumined being.

This illumined being gets its energy directly from the source, God, the universe, the Supreme Being, or whatever you choose to call it. The illumined being is not egotistic and offers a pure form of guidance as they possess extraordinary skills. Their energy is refined, and they can interact with you in a myriad of ways that are suited for you in particular.

The energies they use can be adjusted, and healing will happen in the most efficient manner. More importantly, the illumined individual will always respect your free will and get permission from you before providing any help regardless of what you want. Whether your goal is to improve your Reiki skills or upgrade your healing energy, for instance, the illumined being can help you attain them. If you are already working with a guide, the illumined being can also work closely with them by enabling an upgrade of their skills and improving the quality of their healing energy.

Now, the illumined beings have different names depending on the religious context or the spiritual background of the person seeking their help. Some people call them Jesus; others say that it is Mother Mary, the Holy Spirit, Krishna, Buddha, the Archangels, etc. You may already be utilizing your relationship with any of these illumined beings, but if you don't know how to be in touch with them, the steps below will serve as a guide.

How to Get Help from an Illumined Being

Say a prayer or affirmation

First, you begin by saying a prayer or statement, asking for guidance from the illumined being. This is the first step that you must take after deciding on the illumined nature that you want to work with.

The prayer and affirmation will be the start of the relationship with the illumined being. That will also give you an opportunity to get comfortable with their presence.

Set a time to meditate

You will need to set a particular time during the day that is suitable for meditation. Your times of reflection will help you stay attuned with the illumined being and get used to the unique energy that comes with it.

Pray to the illumined being

At the start of your meditation, pray to the illumined being you have decided to work with so that he or she can make contact with you and strengthen the connection. While praying, you ought to specifically mention the reason why you are reaching out and why you need guidance.

Tell the illumined being that you are passionate about helping others, but you need help in making that happen. At this stage, you should be as open as you can be because every other aspect of this connection will be hinged on what you say in your prayer.

Use the Reiki distance symbol

Next, use the Reiki distance symbol by sending your energy to the illumined being. As you do this, continue with prayers and affirmations; ask the being to work through you and strengthen your energy or connections.

Pray for the illumined being to also enhance your universal energy so that it can be much more effective and beneficial to the individuals you use it on.

Ask for guidance

Ask the illumined being to become your main guide and the main source of your energy. Then, give them permission to heal and make changes within your energy field as it deems fit for your healing.

Right now, you need guidance because others will be coming to you for it. With the illumined being working through you, there is hope of getting support and advice that will enable you to practice Reiki more effectively.

Ask for support

If you are working with guides already, now will also be a good time to ask the illumined body to support and work with them in upgrading their skills and healing energies. You can ask whatever you want in line with Reiki practice, so always feel free to do so in that meditative state.

Remove unhealthy spirits

During the session, you can ask the illumined being to help you get rid of harmful spirits or any other forces that may not be a part of God's plan for you. Now, it is possible that there are negative energies present in your life that affects your Reiki services to recipients.

Ask the illumined being to get the false energies out of your space or environment, too, so that you can practice freely without unnecessary interferences from the wrong vibration.

Use your free will

Illumined beings do not try to exert their will on you; they will always respect your wishes and free will by not forcing anything on you. They will ask permission before making changes with the energy field or providing healing.

Take advantage of this free will and ask for anything else you would like to happen to you or through your Reiki practice. When you make such requests in line with wanting to do good for others, the illumined being will most likely grant your request.

Be guided with your hands

While still in session with the illumined being, place your hands on different parts of your body so that you can appropriate healing there and allow the illumined being's energy to flow through you.

If you have problematic areas or health challenges while praying, use your hands to create contact between your body and the energy from the illumined being. In some cases, you will receive direction on the parts of your body that you should touch, so you should pay attention to what you are doing at all times.

End with a prayer of gratitude

All your sessions with the illumined being should end with a prayer of gratitude and with a request for them to continue helping, guiding, and supporting you with their blessings. You are going to help several other people get better as well, so now is the time to ask for protection from the illumined being and stay grateful for the prayers that you believe are already answered.

You can do this illumined being meditation once daily or as your schedule will allow. It will give you a chance to contemplate this great desire you feel to help others and make the world a better place with Reiki. Remember that this is a very powerful exercise. If you do it continually for a period of years, it will become a huge part of your life.

The illumined being has boundless potentials that can heal you and empower you to do the same for others. Soon enough, they become your only guide (with God, of course). This will quicken your spiritual path while helping your work to get better and better like never before.

It may seem like a process with a lot of steps, but the truth is that if you can get it right within the first few weeks, it will become a part of you long-term. There is so much potential for growth, increased well-being and healing. Still, for you to tap into that potential, you must reach out to a higher authority that can help you create a spiritual pattern.

You cannot succeed with sustaining Reiki if you don't have access to an illumined being. It's like having access to God directly. What can be more potent than that?

Now that you have access to the fundamental aspects of Reiki, always think about getting better and doing better. Look beyond how well you may be doing now and realize that you can do even more if you are dedicated to the process.

The continuation of Reiki is a miracle. It unlocks several doors for you and keeps you inspired. Don't get excited about it once and forget about how well it can affect your life positively later. Just like those kids in Christmas Morning, allow the magic of Reiki to work through you for self-healing and helping others as well.

Well, with this chapter, we can say that we are at the end of our journey, and it has been an exciting one. I believe that you have learned so much about Reiki and that you are ready to implement everything that you know at this point. Concerning implementation, there is a concluding section that you must read as it contains a call to action that will inspire you to utilize the information you have just gained.

Conclusion

Reiki has been used in various forms, and if it has had a long and fruitful history, then it is worth a try. Life will always come at you with varying issues, from the ones you expect to the ones you didn't see coming. Despite the emotional and personal challenges, it is possible for you to overcome them in the most natural way, which is also safe.

Reiki has transcended the level of skepticism and assumptions. We are dealing with a very important healing process that can completely transform your life for good. Hence, in the sections and chapters above, you received extensive details about how to utilize Reiki, as well as other vital information that would make it work for you.

Every human being starts to become concerned about his or her well-being from an early stage in life but being worried about how you feel or the events that cause you to experience imbalanced emotions isn't enough. You must intentionally seek ways to get solutions. That is where Reiki comes into the picture.

In addition to the chapters on ailments and benefits of Reiki, you should also know that Reiki gives a positive boost to your mental health. The #1 topic out there on the internet and everywhere else is the impact of mental health.

If you are wondering why this is the case in 2019, you don't have to anymore because technological disruption enabled a lot of innovations of which social media is at its peak. There are so many people who are completely enthralled by their mobile phones, social media accounts, and the concept of living to impress other people who don't even care about them.

The more involved they are with this circle, the less attention they pay to their mental health, which ultimately leads to a breakdown that could have been avoided. With techniques such as Reiki, one will agree that concerns about mental health can be laid to rest as the well-being of the individual becomes the focus of attention.

Before putting this book down, commit to utilizing Reiki as a self-help practice of protecting your mental health and well-being. It is easier to read a book than implement the details it expresses; this is what separates the people who live well from the one who do not. The former takes action on knowledge gained while the latter does nothing about it.

Remember that Reiki is not an alternative treatment for medical challenges but adjunctive therapeutic support for healing and boosting someone's well-being. If you can get it right with Reiki, then you can get it right with a lot of things mentally, emotionally, and physically.

References

Contessa, L. (2018). 16 Basic Hand position for Self Reiki. Retrieved from https://medium.com/@contessalouise/16-basic-hand-positions-for-self-reiki-c7e19ed6b3f6

Dave, N. (2017). Lifeforce Energy Optimization: How to Experience Transformational Healing. Retrieved from https://www.reikiinfinitehealer.com/lifeforce-energy-optimization

David, H. (2015). Traditional hand positions for Reiki Treatment. Retrieved from https://thereikipage.com/handpos.html

International Association of Reiki Professionals. (2019). Learn about Reiki. Retrieved from https://iarp.org/history-of-reiki/

Indianetzone Reiki, Diseases Cured by Reiki. (n.d.). Retrieved from https://health.indianetzone.com/reiki/1/diseases_cured_by_r eiki.htm

Kathie, L. (n.d.). Distant Healing and the Human Energy Field. Retrieved from https://www.reiki.org/reikinews/distanthealing.htm

Palmer, Miles/ (2011), How to Practice Reiki Self-Treatments. Retrieved from https://reikiinmedicine.org/daily-practice/how-to-practice-reiki-self-treatment/

The Thirsty Soul, Benefits of Reiki. (n.d.) Retrieved from, https://www.thethirstysoul.com/reiki/benefits-of-reiki/

University of Minnesota, What can I Expect in a Typical Reiki Session? (n.d.) Retrieved from https://www.takingcharge.csh.umn.edu/what-can-i-expect-typical-reiki-session